D1581181

The Social Significance of Health Promotion

The Social Significance of Health Promotion sets health promotion in its historical context and delineates its contemporary role. It explores the potential of health promotion to impact on our social values and sense of community.

The book begins by exploring the historical roots of health promotion and its relationship to the medical model of health. It then moves on to present analyses of contemporary health promotion programmes in which the contributors are actively engaged. These chapters discuss current questions for health promotion from a practitioner perspective and from the point of view of their social impact. They cover a wide range of topical issues such as social exclusion and inclusion, the mental health of children, the role of alternative medicine, and health in the workplace.

Emphasising the centrality of empowerment, participation and advocacy to an effective health promotion programme, *The Social Significance of Health Promotion* brings students and professionals right up to date with the latest initiatives and theories.

Théodore H. MacDonald has had a varied and international professional and academic career. He has been a consultant with WHO in the field of Health Promotion and with UNESCO in health and education. He has recently retired from Brunel University, but continues to lecture in the UK and abroad on a freelance basis.

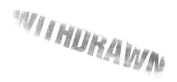

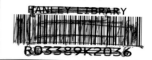

The Social Significance of Health Promotion

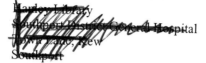

Edited by
Théodore H. MacDonald

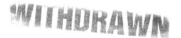

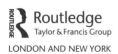 Routledge
Taylor & Francis Group

LONDON AND NEW YORK

First published 2003
by Routledge
11 New Fetter Lane, London EC4P 4EE

Simultaneously published in the USA and Canada
by Routledge
29 West 35th Street, New York, NY 10001

Routledge is an imprint of the Taylor & Francis Group

© 2003 Théodore H. MacDonald

Typeset in Times by Taylor & Francis Books Ltd
Printed and bound in Great Britain by MPG Books Ltd, Bodmin

British Library Cataloguing in Publication Data
A catalogue record for this book is available from the British
Library

Library of Congress Cataloging in Publication Data
The social significance of health promotion/ edited by
Théodore H. Macdonald.
p. cm. Includes bibliographical references and index.
1. Health promotion. 2. Health promotion–Social aspects.
3. Health planning–Social aspects. I. MacDonald, Théodore H.
(Théodore Harney), 1933–
RA427.8.S626 2003
613–dc21

ISBN 0–415–30196–3 (hbk)
ISBN 0–415–30197–1 (pbk)

To all who work to bring about peace and justice – major prerequisites for community health – this book is dedicated.

Contents

Tables

Contributors

Rosie Ayub is lead officer for involvement and consultation with Rochdale Social Services. Her work has involved development of an interagency strategy for consultation and involvement, including a model to bring about change within the organisation and work towards a more fluid and open approach to participation.

Prior to her work in Rochdale she managed an advocacy organisation in Kirklees and worked with a diverse range of people and groups to ensure that people had a voice within the Community Care system. She is committed to working with organisations and individuals to develop more creative and empowering approaches to involvement.

Karen Baistow teaches in the department of Academic Psychiatry, in the Division of Psychological Medicine at King's College, London. Her teaching and research interests lie in the field of mental health, child development and welfare and she has been involved in comparative European research, with particular reference to practice and policy issues in these areas, since the early 1990s. Her current research interests lie in the field of children's mental health promotion. She is the author of a number of journal articles and chapters in edited volumes, and is part-author of two books.

Steven Bell has been Health Promotion Manager with the Highland NHS board since September 2001; he had been Acting Manager since 1999. Previously employed by the Board as a Health Promotion Adviser (1995–9) and as a Community Health Project Co-ordinator in Lochaber (1993–5), Steve also has a background in local government as an elected member of Cleveland County Council (1989–93). He is a contributor to the MSc in Health Promotion at the Robert Gordon University, and is a member of the Course Monitoring Group. He has lectured in Health Promotion for the Open University. He was educated at the University of Teeside (BA (Hons) Social Science) and the University of Glasgow (MPhil, Social Policy/Health Promotion). Currently he is completing an MBA at Glasgow University.

Martha Chinouya is a Post-Doctoral Research Fellow at the University of Surrey. Her doctoral research was devoted to HIV disclosure patterns among affected African families in London. Her research for the National AIDS Trust provides the basis for the Department of Health's HIV policy for African communities. She has instigated innovative health promotion projects based on community-led research funded by NHS Health Authorities and Trusts. These include the Padare Project in Camden and Islington and the Pachedu-Zenzele Action Research Project in London.

Lindsey Dugdill has worked in the field of occupational/workplace health research for over ten years with special interests in health needs assessment, programme development and evaluation. Her work has been implemented within a wide range of organisations in the North West of England, including a variety of organisational types, and sizes, for example, Liverpool City Council, the banking sector and small and medium sized businesses (SMEs). She has collaborated with the Liverpool Occupational Health Partnership for the last decade and has recently co-published an evaluation study on intervention support for health and safety in SMEs. At a national level, she worked for eight years as research adviser and trainer to the Health Education Authority's Health at Work in the NHS programme and also with the Department of Health Workplace Task Force (1992). Internationally, the World Health Organization has published her work on workplace health evaluation (1999–2001). Most recently, she has carried out a large health at work consultation in Sefton, Merseyside with over 200 organisations – 169 being from the small and micro sectors.

Linda Gibson is a lecturer in Public Health at Nottingham. She has an MSc in Health Research from Lancaster University where she is currently completing her doctoral work, which examines the impact of professionalisation on complementary and alternative medicine (CAM). She developed a postgraduate programme in health and social science perspectives of CAM at Liverpool John Moores University, as well as teaching on the undergraduate programme in Health (Studies). She is a founding member of the undergraduate programme in Health Studies. She is also a founding member of the Alternative and Complementary Healthcare Research Network (ACHRN), a forum to support researchers who are doing social science research in CAM in the North West.

Conan Leavey's background is in Social Anthropology and he has made field visits to Zambia to study changes in marriage practices, and then to Kenya as part of a multidisciplinary team investigating oral rehydration therapy use among rural women. As a consequence of this last visit he has developed an interest in how people combine different explanatory systems to make health-related decisions, and how this information can help primary care services meet people's needs more effectively. In 1990, he moved to

Liverpool and completed a PhD on why women in inner city areas do not attend for cervical smears. Subsequently he has worked as a consultant on two other action research projects in primary care and is currently supervising the evaluation of a community arts project with young carers in the Liverpool Health Action Zones. For the last three years he has been working on a British Council-funded link with Tribhvan University in Nepal to develop and evaluate joint research projects in non-formal education. Presently Dr Leavey is the Route Leader for a MSc Health Evaluation Programme – despite his concerns about the whole notion of 'evaluation' in research.

Théodore H. MacDonald, BSc, Med, PhD, MD, has held chairs in medicine, mathematics and education and has in the past ten years established an international reputation as a analyst of global health promotion. As a WHO consultant in some of the world's poorest nations, Professor MacDonald's recent publications focus attention on international fiscal inequities which seriously constrain the implementation of health services in many parts of the world. Recently retired as Director of Postgraduate Studies in Health at Brunel University, Théodore MacDonald is in wide demand as a speaker and adviser on the political and social implications of health promotion policies and public health.

Peter Murray is a writer, researcher and speaker on poverty and health inequalities. He is a former manager of the UK Public Health Association's Poverty and Health Project and has campaigned to raise awareness of Child Health Inequalities. In 1999 he established Scotland's first Children's Rights Project.

He is a member of the 'Free School Meals (Scotland) Bill' campaign group, which seeks universally free and nutritious school meals for all children attending state education. With Dr David Player, he researched and wrote 'The Health of our Children – the Future of our Country', which established the scientific case for the Bill.

Peter Murray is a Social Science Honours Graduate of Glasgow Caledonian University; he is married with two daughters and lives in Glasgow.

Eileen O'Keefe is Senior Lecturer in Philosophy and Health Policy at the University of North London (UNL). Her books address inequalities in health in London and management of community health services within the framework set by the World Health Organization's European Health Strategy. Recent publications are devoted to globalisation, the health impact of World Bank and World Trade Organisation policy, human rights and the mental well-being of children. She co-founded HealthLINK, a network of disabled people to empower their involvement in multi-agency service planning. She manages a British Council-funded Regional Academic Partnership between UNL and the Ukrainian Academy of Public Administration in Odessa. She is a consultant to the Commonwealth Secretariat on the topic of priority-setting in the context of globalisation. She is a member of the American Society of Law Medicines and Ethics.

David Player has had a long career in medicine, qualifying in 1950, and has made a distinguished contribution to public health in the UK, of which he was the co-founder. He served with the Royal Army Medical Corps, in the Far East from 1950 to 1952. A man of vast experience in a wide array of medical specialities, he has been particularly active in the field of mental health. He is especially interested in the welfare of disadvantaged people. For instance, from 1970 to 1973 he was Medical and Psychiatric Adviser to the Secretary of State for Scotland on the Scottish Borstal and Prison Service. He has published in major medical journals.

Jane Springett is Professor of Health Promotion and Public Health, Liverpool John Moores University, and visiting professor at the Institute of Public Health Research and Policy at Salford University. She was a member of the WHO/Euro Working Group on the Evaluation of Health Promotion and currently works with the Pan American Health Organization (PAHO) as a member of the International Evaluation Research Group. She has a background in urban geography and has been involved in research on 'Healthy Cities', focusing particularly on partnerships and intersectoral collaboration. She is currently involved in the evaluation of Manchester Salford and Trafford Health Action Zone and also the Merseyside Health Action Zones. She is committed to participatory action research as a vehicle for change and is working in a number of participatory evaluation projects at the community and policy level.

Rowena Vickridge is Community Care Co-ordinator for Rochdale Social Services and Bury and Rochdale Health Authority. As well as having a strategic policy and planning role she has a lead senior management responsibility for consultation and involvement in community care services.

She has written on collaborative working within health and social care, and has extensive experience of leading change towards joint working at strategic and practice levels, especially in relation to health and social care services for older people. She has had a long-standing interest in developing better ways of supporting the involvement of service users and local communities in service planning and development.

Grahame D. Wright is a lecturer in Health Promotion at the Robert Gordon University in Aberdeen, Scotland. He is also Course Leader for the Master of Science degree in Health Promotion at the institution. Currently he is concerned with analysing how health promotion is mediated in undergraduate curricula of professions allied to medicine. In this respect his particular interest is in programmes for the preparation of physiotherapists, occupational therapists and dieticians. He is strongly of the view that unless the actual teaching in the area of health promotion is community-focused, rather than procedure-driven, its role at the interface between public health and the professional biomedical focus will be seriously compromised.

Preface

A massive change in attitudes to healthcare paradigms began to make itself felt in the West with the coming of age in 1974–1982 of health promotion. Prior to that time, 'health' was pretty well seen as being an objectively measurable phenomenon and the right and proper domain of biomedically trained scientists, principally doctors of medicine in its various tightly defined specialties. As I have shown in various analyses, health promotion was by no means an invention of the 1970s – it has been with us for as long as the history of medicine itself – but the *appreciation* of what its role could be was seriously reconsidered in 1974 (by the signal work of Marc Lalonde) and then this was reinforced and systemised by WHO in 1982.

In order to understand the tone and content of what follows in this book, let me explain what health promotion is and why it now plays the crucial role it does. The very demanding reductionist training required of scientific biomedicine unavoidably created a major 'participation barrier' between clinical practice and the capacity for lay people to make effective and informed use of it. Throughout much of the nineteenth and early twentieth centuries the great medical battles for public health were being fought and won. The refinement of microscopy, for instance, heralded immense strides in bacteriology and the control of specific disease states. Public health was put on a rational and programmatic basis with the development in our great cities of sewerage systems and the like, and with the elaboration of legislation about health and safety in the workplace, food distribution, etc.

But obviously, as major advances were made in scientific medicine, the 'participation barrier' between the healers and the sick became ever greater. Advanced liberal democracies spent increasing proportions of their GNP on improvements to public health, largely by putting more and more funding into the professional biomedical side of the equation until it became obvious (in the 1970s) that such a use of public health money was becoming less efficient in terms of its returns in the form of an increasingly healthy population.

It was only then that questions were seriously considered relating to how the public's use of existing biomedical expertise could be rendered more efficient. Participation had to be re-invigorated. Space does not allow me to deal with the deep and complex philosophical, psychological and sociological aspects thus addressed. Suffice it to say, the issue of 'empowerment' became of pivotal concern. If lay people are really expected to take more responsibility for their health (indeed, some see this as a civic duty, a moral responsibility) they must assume a more equal role in their discourse with health agencies. Among other things, this meant that they had to have real choices. Likewise, the medical providers – doctors, chiropractors, osteopaths, whatever – had to change their attitudes and become much more willing to have their views questioned and challenged by patients.

The scene in Britain today in this respect, is hardly recognizable compared to what it was even as recently as ten or fifteen years ago. In 1987, one of my patients had come to me because of severe insomnia. Initially he simply requested me to give him a script for a certain well-known tranquilliser. I pointed out various objections to such a procedure and explained a few alternatives. I then asked him for his opinion. He looked at me incredulously, and then said: 'But Doc, that's up to you!' Nowadays such a response would be rare. People are much more empowered – sometimes even through TV medical soap-operas – and the media generally are much more liberal with health information (and misinformation).

As far as alternative health approaches are concerned, the situation was quite simple at one time. In 1982, the British Medical Council was categorical in advising orthodox doctors not to get involved in modalities such as homeopathy, acupuncture, etc. But by 1992, their position had changed dramatically and their advice was that GPs needed to be more aware of alternative approaches. Increasingly since then, opportunities for an exchange of views and of methodologies have been encouraged and catered for.

This is all very much a consequence of the empowerment phenomenon mentioned earlier. It is also a consequence of the fact that 'truth' is a slippery fish and can rarely be categorically said to have been established. Increasingly, procedures which have long had the imprimatur of orthodox medicine are going to be questioned. It seems to this writer that this is an irreducible consequence of health promotion and empowerment. It may be exceedingly annoying for some practitioners, who feel more comfortable with a more compliant clientele, but those days are now gone – one hopes.

Health and healthcare are more complex issues now. We know that biomedical clinical factors often are not the dominant determinants of health or disease. Rather more important, often, are the way that people feel about themselves in relation to other people around them, their level of job satisfaction, etc. None of this denigrates the role of biomedicine, but it helps put it into context.

Perhaps this can best be understood in terms of the very positive beneficial impacts of advances in orthodox medicine. Advances in instrumentation have rendered diagnosis much more accurate nowadays than we could have hoped for even twenty years ago. On the one hand, our populations in the metropolitan nations are becoming healthier and healthier, widening still further the participation gap between people who are ill and the people treating them. Biomedicine's remit is not health but illness. Healthy people must feel empowered to choose – and such a level of empowerment may well not lead them into the care of people whose remit is illness rather than health! Biomedicine quite properly may have much less impact in mediating health than it ever has had in its long and distinguished history. And when it does address health issues – rather than specific disease phenomena – it has to be ready to contend with other voices, other points of view. The once magisterial priority of biomedicine, as an arbiter of healthcare has some-times now been usurped by other modalities to which many people feel access is more comfortable.

We have to be ready to discuss. In no science is 'truth' easy to establish, but in the health sciences it is much more difficult because people feel much more involved with what is right or wrong with their health than they would be, say, about the expanding universe versus other models of it. Unquestionably, many orthodox medical practitioners might feel outraged that what seems patently obvious to them, and to be well backed up by statistics, can be ques-tioned. And to the extent that they refuse to tolerate even the discussion of other points of view, they weaken the degree to which their scientific training can be of much use in the shifting empowerment equations of lay people.

It is my hope that the present book will inform and stimulate the discourse further by focusing attention on the social significance of health promotion – its impact, for instance, on civic society, social norms and values, connected-ness among and between groups of people and on their perception and practice of health. With this in mind, an immensely variegated group of eminent practitioners working in the front line of health promotion, have agreed to contribute reflections and analyses of their own strategies in addressing the social significance issue. The book is intended to provide prac-tical guidance, backed up by hands-on experience. To contextualise all of this activity, three of the contributors analyse the historical perspective in detail.

Théodore H. MacDonald
London, July 2002

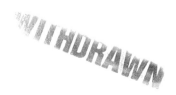

Acknowledgements

Let me say at the outset that it would be well nigh impossible to thank by name all of the people who have made this book possible. No doubt my fellow contributors are similarly indebted to other unnamed people and agencies. In my case, for instance, I owe thanks to Dr Sebastian Garman, one of my former colleagues at Brunel University. His general support is appreciated and, in particular, he provided editorial assistance with one of the chapters.

Vanessa Winch, Production Editor for Routledge, was of great assistance, especially in the final stages of the book's preparation. It also goes without saying that I extend most grateful thanks to the contributors, whose names and details are to be found immediately after the contents. I also extend special thanks to Barbara Lee for much of the clerical and keyboard work involved, and to Conor Gissane for his computer wizardry, especially with respect to complicated diagrams.

Finally, I cannot possibly forget to mention my wife, Chris, and our son, Matthew, whose love and forbearance helped enormously to keep the project going.

Chapter 1

Ancient epistemological bases for health promotion

Théodore H. MacDonald

This chapter will initially confront the reader with some of the epistemological problems underlying the understanding of the origins of health promotion. In particular, it will deal with the attitudes and provenances for them that may have undergirded ancient views on health, its bases and promotion.

After dealing with the issue of reductionism, the reader will be introduced to belief systems about health, length of life, the idea of some previous golden age when people were not prey to ill health, attitudes engendered by these belief systems and models of healthcare to which they gave rise. To reduce the compass of such a vast undertaking, emphasis will be placed principally on developments in the Western context, although references to other ethnic contexts will be included, both to encourage broader reading around the issues and to indicate common themes.

The cardinal role played by the 'goddesses' Panacea and Hygieia as symbols of the two different approaches to health that continue to be represented in modern international clinically based healthcare on the one hand and health promotion on the other, is analysed at length. The chapter closes with a challenge to consider health promotion's role in possibly over-sanitizing the world in which we live.

Science, myth and health promotion

Science, as a system of thought and inquiry, has freed us and has empowered us – as individual people and as entire societies – in ways too numerous to detail. Historically, the dominance of the scientific method in human affairs has been of comparatively recent provenance, even in the Western world. Also, this has been a gradual process, beginning with some Egyptian and Meso-potamian thinkers not much earlier than 1500 BC – a gradual process that didn't really take off in a big way in Europe until the Renaissance. The leitmotif of scientific progress though, has been the rigorous refinement of 'reduc-tionism' as a strategy of thinking since the time of Isaac Newton. It is important to understand this clearly if we are to make any sense of the devel-opment of health studies and of health promotion.

Reductionism is best appreciated in its simplest expression in mathematics. If we can narrow down ('reduce', hence 'reductionism') the focus of our inquiry to the actions of two variables – one independent (x) and one dependent (y), so that we can write an equation.

$$y = f(x)$$

(or 'y is some defined function of x'), it not only means that a given value of x will determine the value of y, but that we can *experiment* with different values of x to discover truths about the nature of y.

Thus, the power of reductionism as a strategy depends on trying to get down to the point at which, ideally, we are only working on two variables at a time, or, at the very least, can ascertain which are dependent and independent variables. Outside of mathematics, this is often excruciatingly difficult to achieve. Moreover, when we are dealing with health, the confounding factors are numerous.

For instance, an important 'myth' in the modern development of health as a focus for scientific inquiry is the account of Koch and his discovery of the link between bacteria and disease. At this point it is important for the reader to try to recall what he or she knows about Robert Koch and his research work on bacteria. What he actually did and saw are, if you like, his 'story' (or even better, 'history'), while how it is told and the meaning attached to it, constitute the 'myth'. Myths in science! Surely not! But let us see.

Suppose you have forgotten what Koch's contribution was, and have had to look it up in some 'neutral' source such as an encyclopaedia. The following is an extract from the account given in Compton's Encyclopaedia of 1997. I have numbered the sentences for later analysis.

1   Robert Koch (1843–1920) was a German country doctor who helped to raise the study of microbes to the modern science of bacteriology.
2   By painstaking laboratory research, he showed how specific microbes cause specific diseases.
3   His wife bought him a microscope for his twenty-eighth birthday, which he immediately began to use to study anthrax microbes.
4   He raised cultures of anthrax and injected these into healthy animals.
5   They developed anthrax.
6   He proved that animals with anthrax had these microbes, while healthy ones did not.
7   Also he showed that, once an animal had been given anthrax by injection, it began to produce anthrax microbes and these could be used to infect other animals.
8   In subsequent years he similarly isolated the tubercle bacillus and showed that it was not present in healthy animals but only in tubercular ones.
9   Later on he also isolated the cholera bacillus.

Told in this way, the Koch story reflects a desire for a dependable reductionist view of health. Find out what causes the disease – hopefully only one agent – learn to identify it, eliminate it and thus cure the patient of the disease in question. It does not behove us to make light of the 'reductionist myth' in the development of health care and of healthier communities. Those of us who work in medicine and health-related areas owe a huge debt to those 'microbe hunters' of the nineteenth and twentieth century. But there are at least two aspects of the simple reductionist view that need to be thought about more deeply. The first is to be clear about what we mean by 'health'. Is health just the absence of disease, such that if we successfully target and eliminate each disease, we will have health? Then, second, in the Koch story – as relayed in the encyclopædia account – can we separate the story from the myth? Let us try, sentence by sentence.

For instance, sentence No. 2 is a little worrying. Koch never claimed to show how a bacillus caused the disease in question, but only that those particular types of bacilli were present in animals with that particular disease.

Moreover, sentence No. 2 leaves us with a level of reductionist certainty to which we have no right. If we could get rid of all TB bacilli, we would not have to contend with TB as a disease but TB bacilli do not always, not even usually, cause their human hosts to develop tuberculosis. One has to be infected with the relevant bacillus to develop TB, but only a small percentage of those so infected actually become ill with TB. There must be other factors. Most readers of this book are hosts to colonies of the TB bacillus but remain healthy. What then are we to make of sentence No. 6, for is it also a fact that not all animals that are hosts to anthrax bacilli have the disease? Similarly, sentences Nos 8 and 9 need closer scrutiny. The reader can easily find other concerns in the account given. Many other caveats will emerge throughout this chapter.

Using the reductionist approach to TB control, we made great strides in eliminating that scourge in both Europe and North America. But parallel with all the mass chest X-ray programmes and TB testing, other non-medical developments were accruing. Sewerage engineering ensured cleaner streets and homes, housing legislation began to be passed as did legislation about working conditions in industry. This all created a huge range of factors that struggling reductionists could not hope to handle. For instance, legislation relating to food purity or housing most certainly had a direct impact on public health, but such factors also gave people a greater sense of autonomy and self-worth. We know statistically that illness is less likely to strike down people with high self-esteem. It has even been shown that people 'who are actively religious are less likely to become ill' (Astrow et al., 2001: 287).

Clearly health is not only the absence of disease, but relates to social and political factors which fall well outside the conventional reductionist approach. This does not in any way denigrate reductionism, the epistemological basis of the scientific method, but it means that people who are concerned with health promotion have to learn to deal with a huge array of uncertainties, social and political values, belief systems and philosophical issues which may seem at first to be only remotely connected to the health sciences. As will become evident to the reader, these philosophical issues are also basic to what the author calls 'informed empowerment' and that, in turn, is the pivot on which health promotion turns.

Applying scientific methods to health

As people, we are aware of an 'external world', replete with phenomena such as gravity, weather, rock formations, plants and other animals, etc. Although our progress towards understanding such phenomena has by no means been smooth, with frequent evidence of people slipping back into superstition, it has been exponentially gaining ground throughout the world for the last 300 years or so. The same is also true, but to a much more limited extent, when it comes to our awareness of our 'internal world' – the phenomena of life, health, illness, death, consciousness, etc.

Myths from almost every known culture show that people have found it extremely difficult to accept that the 'internal' and 'external' worlds are not, somehow, qualitatively different. A craving for immortality did not impede Isaac Newton's efforts to draw up a model of how the physical world worked. But when it came to his own body and health, and those of other people, he was more than prepared to accept, without question, the teachings of the Church. Most English-speaking readers will be aware of some of these teachings and the content of the first five chapters of the Book of Genesis in the Bible will doubtless be familiar to many. According to that account, humans were created as 'different' from the rest of the universe as being in 'the image of God'. If Eve had not let her curiosity run away with her, we humans would have never left the Garden of Eden. Even after being expelled from there, succeeding generations of people were convinced that there had been in some unidentified distant past, a golden age, when people (because they lived innocently in a state close to nature) were comparatively free of disease and lived for extraordinary lengths of time, for example, Methusulah (Gen. 5), Jared, etc. Even Noah is reported to have lived to be 500 years old, and – compared with the others referred to in that chapter – he died comparatively early!

As far back as 1000 BC, a similar Greek mythology was well established. This involved a golden age followed by a silver and a bronze age, each successively less glorious than its predecessor, in which people were much bigger, healthier and longer-lived than people are now. We find similar mythologies in various non-Western cultures.

From all of this, many people have tended to develop a rather dualistic approach to science and health. All phenomena not directly related to our 'inner world' can freely be investigated by reductionist scientific techniques, but when it comes to issues like disease, mortality and immortality, people often see themselves as different from other natural phenomena.

The golden age belief is not hard to find among Western people living sophisticated lives today in our great cities. Many alternative health modalities emphasise the 'back to nature' theme. Indeed, without these ideas, it would be difficult to account for the content of much great music, art and writing. To draw attention to this rather awkward fact does not necessarily invalidate such belief systems, but it is important that health promoters be aware that to be ignorant of such phenomena must reduce their capacity to work effectively at the interface between reductionist clinical science and people's non-reductionist experience of healthy living in the community. Many able and responsible scientifically trained people swear by organic food – with perhaps an equally impressive group opposing it – but to the average lay-person, the appeal is not to scientific rigour but to the 'back to nature' myth, the yearning for a past golden age which probably never existed. Sciences dealing with the 'external world' are relatively free from such 'golden age' mythology.

In the Greek context, the first real attempt to look at health in scientific terms was that of Hippocrates (c. 460–370 BC). The science of the day taught that there were four elements – earth, air, fire and water – and that everything was derived from these. Figure 1.1 shows how, even prior to Hippocrates, the Greeks had linked this basic belief about the physical world with a model of how health might work. Note the corners of the inner square, containing the four elements. Fire is both hot and dry, and water is moist and cold. Earth can be cold or dry and air can be moist or hot. Summer (on the Peloponnesian peninsula) is hot and dry, autumn is cold and dry, winter moist and cold and spring moist and hot. These attributes were associated with the four 'biles' or 'humours', which Hippocrates regarded as mediating health by the extent to which they were 'balanced'.

If one is not well, then the humours are not appropriately balanced. If black bile (associated with the spleen) dominates, then the person will suffer from disorders which Hippocrates called melancholia (*melan* = black, *cholia* = bile). Too much white bile leads to phlegmatism (apathy, lethargy), too much red bile leads to disorders characterised by a sanguine (courageous, passionate) disposition, while too much yellow bile and biliousness refers to liver upsets.

Such a model immediately suggests a possible logical response to various illnesses, although obviously the appropriateness or otherwise of such interventions depended ultimately on how accurate the initial model was. But it was a great step forward and will be dealt with further in this chapter. Contrast it with Egyptian medical epistemology. The Egyptians were very advanced in certain surgical interventions. For instance, they carried out operations involving brain tumour removal and became amazingly expert at surgical techniques requiring making holes (fenestrations) in the cranium to gain access. But they had no systematic observation-based approach to a science of health and disease (Singer *et al.* 1962). They explained the world in terms of gods. Priests were the healers or medical men because they communicated with the gods. Ideas about the body and its health were largely analogical, without as much

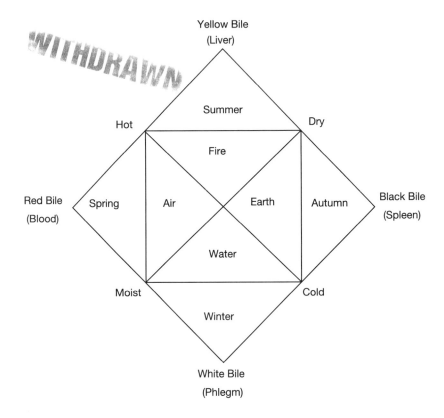

Figure 1.1 The Hippocratic conception of the link between disease, the four
       seasons and the four elements

epistemological basis as later characterised Greek speculation. For instance, the
Egyptians tended to think of the body as being like the River Nile in that it
could become blocked. To get 'unblocked', one took laxatives, induced vomit-
ing or had 'bad blood' sucked out by black leeches (Singer *et al.* 1962).

Oriental medical foundations, though beyond the remit of this chapter,
are also rich in interest. For instance, the yin and yang idea is not unlike the
Greek four-element model and could be tied in with health, the four seasons
and the weather in much the same way.

In all of this, it is not difficult to recognise the 'back to nature' resonance
of the golden age idea. As people were supposedly bigger, healthier, longer-
lived, more god-like the further back you went, a bias still persists that the
'closer to nature' one can get, the healthier one will be. Much of the New
Age movement and of alternative health belief is governed by this idea.

People working in health promotion are especially subject to such belief
systems, even if only unconsciously. Indeed, well before Hippocrates' time,

Greek mythology, had developed a story-line for accommodating two rather opposite approaches to healthcare – one based on a top-down interventional and physician-directed modality and the other based on a lifestyle, holistic and self-directed modality. It is not hard for the reader to appreciate the similarity between a strongly clinically based, interventionist, consultancy-directed bio-medicine on the one hand and a more user-friendly, indeed sometimes amateur, combination of health promotion and local advocacy approaches based on 'empowerment'.

What is instructive is the way the Greeks, especially from the time of Hippocrates, tried to separate the two and to draw on a combination of reli-gious myths and common sense to do so. The basic story is very ancient, probably dating back to 1500 BC at least.

Health promotion prefigured in Ancient Greece

The present author has argued in a previous publication (MacDonald 1998) that Greek mythology did actually provide the medical practitioners of the day with a dual option, allowing an emphasis on interventionist medical care on the one hand and an emphasis on how individuals and communities could lead health-affirming lives on the other. Almost 1,000 years before Hippo-crates, the prevailing health belief among ancient Peloponnesian people was that illness was a punishment inflicted on them by the god Apollo. The only solution was (very much along the Egyptian lines already referred to) to make supplication to Apollo. But, as ill-health became increasingly the focus of a more philosophically analytical mind-set, the supplicatory religious framework gradually gave way to a system in which the 'deities' worked through rational channels, almost as aids to human effort. Hippocrates, in his *Diagnostics* (Jones 1945, vol. 7: 388) as far back as about 400 BC, even makes the comment that 'although we invoke the gods by name and pray to them, the physician knows that they are not real beings, but ways of describing what we have learned by observation to be true'.

One of the gods invoked to provide a more user-friendly approach in contrast to a purely supplicatory approach was Aesclepius, supposedly Apollo's son. The story is that, before becoming a god, Aesclepius lived as a mortal on earth, where he learned the art of healing from a centaur named Chiron. Aesclepius applied this new-found knowledge so liberally that people started to live increasingly long lives and he was even said to have raised people from the dead. Hades, god of the underworld, complained to Zeus about the lack of recruits entering his domain in the afterlife. Zeus addressed the issue by striking Aesclepius dead with a thunderbolt. But, of course, this action of Zeus angered Apollo and, to appease Apollo, Zeus elected Aesclepius to become the god of medicine.

Now Aesclepius, while a mortal on earth, had two daughters, Panacea and Hygieia. Both had worked with Aesclepius in his mortal embodiment with Panacea preparing herbal remedies and the like for specific illnesses, while her sister, Hygieia, concentrated on advising people on how to live healthy and fulfilling lives. It is from Panacea's name, of course, that the expression 'panacea' is derived, and from the name of Hygieia we derive the concept of 'hygiene' or 'public health'. In time, both Panacea and Hygieia themselves became goddesses of health and, even prior to Hippocrates' time, medical practitioners tended to specialise, either as Panaceists or Hygieaists. In one exchange with an apprentice doctor, Thrasymachus, in the *Diagnostics*, Hippocrates explains that 'Diseases of the soul' (what we now call 'mental illness') fall outside the remit of panacaeists and should be dealt with by devotees of Hygieia. If Hippocrates really did make such a comment (we have no way of knowing), or even if it was made by someone anxious to establish, posthumously, the credentials of the great man, it is indeed a wise and seminal statement. It recognises mental illness as a legitimate focus of medicine. It also recognises that 'good health', either mental or physical, is not exclusively a matter for a reductionist and purely deterministic approach, but also must involve recognition that a person's relationship to him/herself and to his/her social milieu and physical environment are also important. In other words, as any good health promoter would say today, 'empowerment is the key to a high standard of community health'.

A reading, even a most cursory one, of the history of medicine suggests that these two polarities have governed medical practice and our understanding of health and disease ever since. What we now refer to as 'alternative' modalities of healthcare (e.g. Homeopathy, Herbalism, Iris Diagnosis, etc) tend to reflect Hygieia-type values, while orthodox medicine remains largely under Panacea-type influences. At some points in our history, the two modalities have been very separate and at other times they have been very close. For instance, in the West in the 1960s and 1970s, such great strides were being made in orthodox biomedicine, that alternative modalities were very much marginalised. This was especially so in America.

But then, by the mid-1980s, the calls from the ranks of orthodox medicine to ban alternative modalities became less strident. In 1992 the British Medical Council released a statement saying that 'doctors must learn to co-operate', insofar as they could without compromising orthodox belief and practice, with alternative practitioners. Throughout the late 1980s and early 1990s, there were drives to register certain alternative health systems and to give them equal status with orthodox medicine. But if one goes back to 1982, the British Medical Council issued a statement to GPs declaring that any modalities other than the orthodox ones were best avoided (MacDonald, 1996: 279).

As stated before, this has gone on throughout the history of Western medicine. It is important, therefore, for the reader to appreciate that, just because the phrase 'health promotion' was not in use much before Lalonde's use of it in 1974 (MacDonald 1998: 11) this does not mean that the ideas which govern and sustain the values implicit in health promotion are modern. They are almost as old as scientific, interventionist medicine, as we shall now indicate. The next section will look at the impact of this, as the author considers how, and to what extent, primitive health beliefs have formed a basis for the development of modern health beliefs in Western culture.

Social and political contexts for development of rational health beliefs

Primitive peoples' speculations upon life must have been influenced by the required 'mode of life' or set of 'survival strategies' in various contexts. But common to all of these would surely be this. One of the first things that induced people to reflect on life, either religiously or analytically, must have been the fact of death. Observations of the actual course of death led to important physiological insights. People learned to observe heartbeat and it is not difficult to see how, in almost all primitive cultures, the heart became regarded as the seat of life. Likewise, experiences in battle (or in the slaughter of animals) gave rise to the belief that the head is rather vital (!) and that blood flows around the body. Indeed, one of the principal descriptive motifs in Homer's *Iliad* is not simply that people were killed in battle, but prolonged descriptions of how: where, say, the spear penetrated and details of the death throes.

Again, the deep expiration which so often signals the moment of death, almost certainly gave rise to the idea of life having something to do with the nature of air. It also drew attention to its dependence on the lungs and their rhythmical movements. This is such a primitive idea that we can have no way of tracing its origins. One not only finds the God of Genesis, breathing the breath (spirit) into lifeless models of people, but ancient Sanskrit writings, pre-dating the Genesis accounts, reflect the same basic idea. Doubtless the concept of immortality, which did not trouble scientists dealing with phenomena in the natural world, arose from the idea that the breath (spirit) of life leaves the dead person but continues to live independently of the corpse In ancient Greek, the word *pneuma* (from which of course, we get the words 'pneumatic' and 'pneumonia') referred to both 'breath' and 'spirit'. We shall deal more fully with this concept in the next section.

Moving a step further, we can see that it was natural for people to try to 'fix' defective bodily machines to forestall death. Primitive surgery would have derived from such situations. As to naturally occurring fatal disease, rather than death by injury in battle, the response at first was no doubt less analytical because the causes were that much less visible and immediate. This allowed a parallel development of supplicatory and superstitious beliefs, which set a limit to the natural exercise of attempts to 'understand'. However, over time it became obvious that many fatal diseases follow pretty specific courses. Again, the Greeks came to our rescue here.

Bubonic plague devastated the city of Athens in 430–31 BC. Because the Greeks were such prodigious chroniclers, we have many written accounts of these events and they became less and less interested in superstition and reference to gods, and more analytical as time passes. The description given by Thucydides in his account of the Peloponnesian War is surprisingly 'modern' in his stalwart refusal to entertain superstition and his stated effort to be guided only by accurate descriptors of epidemiological phenomena (Thucydides 1966). This sort of thing is the bedrock from which, over the intervening centuries, our current ideas about pathology, morbidity and physiology have developed.

Together with this, of course, theories of pharmacology were developed, because the panaceists were always prescribing various regimens for disease states. It seems apparent that it was the gradual change in the balance between supplicatory superstitions and attempts to sort issues out rationally that really caused the Hippocratic system to assume hegemony as the first 'scientific' approach to health. In every society, the essential 'imperviousness' of fatal diseases made them a focus of religious superstition, and it was natural for 'doctors' at first to be 'successful intercessors' with the gods. Some societies took much longer than did the Greeks to gradually break away from this. The priesthood of the superstitionists had no particular reason to discuss their techniques, because ultimately they were based on magic and supplication. But doctors relying on a process of coming to conclusions on the basis of direct observation would rely very heavily on conversation, both with the patient and with other practitioners. Evidence of this is legion in fifth-century BC Greek literature.

This is not to imply a sharp epistemological chasm between the Greeks and their intellectual forebears – the other peoples of the East, the Egyptians, Persians, Babylonians, etc. To describe the insights of these people would turn this chapter into an entire book, but one terribly important fact should be borne in mind. These previous civilizations may have had the intellectual ability to move from superstition to rationalism, but they did not have the social apparatus. Only the Greeks had been making a systematic effort to create a participatory democracy, in which, because the people played a large role in determining their laws and their leadership, it was natural for them to expect accountability. That kind of social structure did not accommodate well to mute acceptance of state-sanctioned superstition. If nothing else, this illustrates the empowerment aspect of health promotion, based on people's understanding of who they are and how they interact with their environment – social and national.

A recently modern reminder of this – if one is needed – is the role of Trofim D. Lysenko in the former Soviet Union. Science cannot be independent of its social context. It just cannot flourish as well in totalitarian contexts. To make effective ideological use of Lysenko, most of the leading Russian geneticists had to be eliminated. The lucky ones fled to the West, where they flourished. While genetics went from strength to strength in the West, it gradually fell far behind in the East – victim of a 'priesthood', as it were, and of the perceived need to maintain an orthodoxy based on ideology rather than on dispassionate observation.

While there is insufficient space to go into these crucial developments in detail, it is important to examine the processes by which Greek medicine so dramatically developed a rationalist basis. To do this, let us return to its origins in superstition and religion.

A brief analysis of earlier Greek medical sciences

As we have already seen, the earliest beginnings of medical insight among the Greeks, as in all other primitive peoples, were rooted in superstition. For instance, the myth about Aesclepius and his two daughters, Hygieia and Panacea, were firmly anchored in the religious tradition. But it was not long before attempts to make rational sense of the 'four elements/four humours' model secularised the Aesclepian priesthood. It seems reasonable to infer that it probably happened as follows. We know that near the more famous temples to Aesclepius hospitals were built. These attracted large numbers of patients, some of whom might have really been ill, but many of whom were hypochondriacs. For the former group, it was pretty well hit or miss. Either they would recover through natural causes and not through Aesclepian techniques, or they would die. But the fame and glory of Aesclepian medicine would have been spread by the hypochondriacs. The very necessity of having to watch over the course of diseases in these hospitals created a good source of empirical knowledge. In time, a class of purely secular healers, drawing on all of this data, gradually found themselves better able to predict the course of many diseases than the priests could.

One of the largest of these Aesclepian hospitals was at Epidauros in Greece, and today records of the centre can still be consulted there. From about 525 BC onward, these records reflect a definitely more analytical than religious approach in describing the symptoms of arriving patients, and there is evidence that, while some of the religious and superstition-based practices persisted in the temple itself, such as the use of snakes to 'kiss' the affected body part, rationally based interventionist treatments were used in the hospital itself. A century or so earlier, the Aesclepians founded a private guild whose members were bound by a Code of Ethics, which trainee physicians had to swear before being allowed to practise. Among the tenets of this oath were that he (only males were allowed):

- pledged to help his teachers and his professional colleagues;
- to give free medical instruction to the sons of other practitioners and to freely share any new medical discoveries;
- to heal the sick as effectively as possible;
- not to mix or administer poison;
- to refrain from inducing abortions.

Not only do these aims reflect a distinctly rational and non-superstitious approach, but they bear a striking resemblance to what is currently known as the Hippocratic Oath, which most modern doctors have to swear before qualifying (Singer *et al.* 1962: 178).

The ancient records preserve the names of seven notable physicians named 'Hippocrates'. The one who has been called the Father of Medicine and who is credited with emphasising a rational approach to illness, based on meticulous case history taking and observation of symptoms and a rejection of treatment modalities drawn from tradition without evidence of effectiveness, was born on the island of Cos into a family of Aesclepian physicians. Having studied Aesclepian medicine under his father, he was sent to Athens in his late adolescence to study philosophy.

His fame in medical science is due not only to his insistence that the gods were but figures of speech and that in medicine we must be guided only by evidence and good case histories, but also by the fact that he published prolifically, a strategy which he learned in the atmosphere of intellectual ferment in Athens. There is considerable doubt now, however, about how much of what is still published under his name is really his or was interpolated by later hagiographers. Of the entire *Corpus Hippocraticum* (Jones 1945, vol. 7: 415–37), only a few sections are now regarded as his (Bellamy and Pfister 1992: 35). The treatise 'Airs, Waters and Places' (Section II of Jones's 1945 translation) is, however, universally accepted as his own and reflects his brilliant use of the four elements, the four humours and the four seasons. In that treatise we also first run across Hippocrates' views on the four 'humours' and how they link to the four 'elements'. He notes that when blood is allowed to coagulate, it separates into four components: black clots (melan), red viscous residue (red bile), serum (yellow bile) and fibrin (phlegm). He incorporated the element of fire as pneuma, or life-giver or soul. His views on the links of this paradigm with the seasons was based on years of observation and case histories in which he noted a relationship between the sorts of ailments which afflicted people at different times of year.

What is evident is that much of his understanding of anatomy and of physiology was based on dissection of animals. Human dissection was generally avoided because of a lingering belief in ghosts. This led to many errors. For instance, when a mammal is slaughtered – because when the jugular is cut arterial blood drains away – its left ventricle tends to empty out while the right one fills. Examination of the hearts of recently slaughtered mammals led

Hippocrates to conclude that only the right side of the heart dealt with blood, while the left side pumped air through the system as a coolant.

He had very little idea of the nervous system, confusing larger nerves with tendons and seeing the brain as a gland which segregated water, cooled the blood and collected mucus from the body. The mucus was then discharged through the nose. However, he also regarded it as obvious – from reports of death in battle – that the brain must be also the centre of thought and feeling. Within a few years of Hippocrates' death, the idea of the brain mediating mucus flow was dropped.

Space does not permit me to go into further detail about Hippocrates and his 'school', but before moving on to medieval and Renaissance ideas which are now reflected in health promotion, it is vital to make the reader aware of a few crucial aspects of Hippocrates' influence.

1   He reflected a clear awareness that, while individual diseases had a 'course' of development which, if studied carefully, might show ways of arresting them, the actual causes of disease were usually more complex than that.
2   Although he did not believe in divine powers as such, he saw in the Hygieia and Panacea deities convenient figures of speech for the rational promotion of good health and the cure of individual diseases. This represents clear evidence that, although the term 'health promotion' was not used until Lalonde did so in 1974 (Lalonde 1974: 31), the concept has been there all along, since the very beginnings of rationally based medicine.
3   In 'Airs, Waters and Places' (Jones 1945, vol. 3: 415–37), his famous treatise on the effect of seasons and environment on health, Hippocrates emphasised the importance and scope of the Hygieia aspects.
4   Although his anatomy and physiology was often incorrect, his stress on the need to study these carefully led the way to his school of medicine making rapid advances subsequently.
5   In all, the Hippocratic school, itself derived from the Aesclepian priesthood, remained dominant until Alexandrian times c. AD 350. That means that Hippocratic medicine held sway in Western culture for close on 800 years. If we date modern medicine from, say, AD 1457 (Vesalius), this would mean that it has not yet lasted as long as the Hippocratic tradition.

There is much more that can be said about the details of post-Hippocratic developments in health science up until the final demise of the Hippocratic school. For instance, with the development of extensive trading links between Athens and Asia in the east, and Italy in the west, Hippocratic medicine did not remain an exclusively Greek phenomenon but took root in a variety of cultures each with their own primitive 'health discourse'.

This meant that, in the case of Western civilization it constituted a pivotal influence and provided a basis for Europe's rapid developments in scientific medicine, along with an awareness of public health (Hygieia's influence again) as part of its Renaissance after the Dark Ages. It is not within the remit of this chapter to detail the history of modern health promotion, but rather to establish a basis for insight into its development.

I will therefore finish this chapter with a wide-ranging survey of how the reductionist view of conquering individual pathogens fitted in with the growing awareness of public health in Europe up to the modern age.

Public health versus individual disease

When an individual becomes gravely ill, the people around him or her observe the onset and development and, presumably, hope it doesn't it happen to them. In such a situation, it is easy to see why these individual episodes were regarded as some kind of divine punishment, because it is never difficult to recall the particulars of an individual's wrong-doing! The issue becomes more problematical with large-scale epidemics. For instance, Defoe's *Diary of the Plague Year*, which first appeared in 1722, is well worth the attention of any health promoter in this regard. In that book, Defoe describes as a journalist, the bubonic plague epidemic as it affected England in 1665. Indeed, the various 'Black Death' epidemics that ravaged Europe from the 1300s to the 1600s provide prime examples of the way people respond differently to an epidemic than they do to individual fatal illnesses.

For one thing, the situation is much more likely to be chronicled, and this alone makes it more likely that at least some rational analysis will be applied to it. However, such plagues can also reinvest anti-scientific thought with a new legitimacy. One reason for this is that all such epidemics tend to follow a course best exemplified by the sigmoid curve (see Figure 1.2).

At A, a small number of people are infected. By droplet infection, and similar mechanisms, the number of infected people increases (B). Once (B) has reached a sizeable number, each individual spreading the disease to others rapidly, its advance takes on an exponential character, until all of the people who are susceptible out of that population have become infected (C). From then on, the rate at which people are dying decreases because there are fewer and fewer disease-ridden people left (D). After that, the epidemic ends abruptly because there are no more susceptible people left to infect and die (F).

The actual length of time it takes for the plague to run its course in a given population naturally varies. Such factors vary with the actual disease, the population size, etc., but it is never very long. In practice, this means that almost any means generated by the affected population to stop the plague will seem to work.

A very well-known example of this is provided by the situation in and around the small German town of Oberammergau near Munich. In 1633, the village found itself in the path of the spreading bubonic plague epidemic. Under the leadership of the Church, the people of Oberammergau were

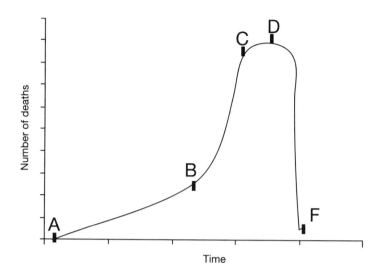

Figure 1.2 The sigmoid curve model of a serious epidemic disease

persuaded, as part of their appeal for divine assistance, to promise to put on a play every ten years, depicting the last week of Christ's life on Earth. By 1634, the necessary levels of organisation had been set up and the play was held. It worked – the plague ended! That play has been held every ten years (except for 1948) in gratitude ever since (Bentley 1984).

As we have observed before, rational and analytical responses are more easily focused on the course of a single disease in individuals; but this tends to focus too specifically on purely reductionist thinking, to the exclusion of more broadly based social and environmental analogues. For instance, the doctrine of a specific aetiology for each disease-state had immense impact during the nineteenth century in the West and seemed to be a universal winner. The history of public health in the West during that period can be read in triumphalist terms, with one disease after another falling to the patient research of microscopists and doctors. As we saw in discussing Robert Koch's work at the beginning of this chapter, some disease states could (it seems) be produced experimentally by infecting healthy animals with pathogens. This idea quickly spread and seemed to provide the ideal, if not the only legitimate *vade mecum*, for exploring and understanding disease. Not only bacteria, but vitamin deficiencies, hormonal imbalances and various physiological stresses came to be regarded as specific causes of specific diseases. Hygieia seemed to shrink into the background as Panacea took centre stage and the idea that somehow lifestyles, one's religious predilections and other social and political factors might be relevant seemed obscure and not worthy of serious scientific study.

There can be no question but that the idea of specific aetiologies provided an immense boost to the authority of scientific medicine. But now, in the twenty-first century, we realise that it has provided a complete account of the cause and course of disease in very few cases. Various cancers elude such approaches, as do conditions such as mental diseases, arteriosclerosis, rheumatic diseases and many others. One view, current among many medical researchers, is that this is entirely because of lack of data. There is a reductionist answer to everything but it is just that we don't yet know enough! In the very long term, presumably, we should be able to account from A to Z for everything from mumps to Beethoven's Ninth Symphony – provided nothing disastrous happens to us first, such as a rogue meteor colliding with Earth or an innocent-looking 'flu virus suddenly wiping us all out.

But that is hopefully a long way off. Health promotion finds itself working in a huge field between known specific aetiologies (and research on others) and the complex interplay between politics, sociology, psychology and people's attempts to seek fulfilment and joy. The specific aetiologists must continue their researches, but as health promoters we also know that most disease states are the indirect outcome of a constellation of circumstances and that these are a proper focus of non-clinical considerations as well as the direct result (sometimes) of single determinant factors.

We acknowledge that the search for the one cause of a specific disease has led to a wider public health movement emphasising decent housing, sewerage, cleanliness, etc. We also must acknowledge, though, that these measures did not spring exclusively – or even principally – from the efforts of the microbe hunters, but from a growing awareness of the rights of people. The Industrial Revolution, which in Britain between 1760 and about 1832 gradually crowded people into cities in unsafe and insanitary conditions, led to phenomena such as the rapid expansion of an awareness of individual rights, and this, in turn, was paralleled by the growth of phenomena like Wesleyism (with its emphasis on individual accountability), trade unionism, etc. A rather good analogy is provided by Réné Dubos in his book *Mirage of Health* (1960: 20), when he points out that while pouring water on a fire tends to solve that problem, no one would suggest that fire is caused by lack of water!

Indeed, I would like to close this chapter with an even more provocative suggestion, drawn from another well-known public health tale. The reader has doubtless heard of John Snow, who is famous in another context, that is, the use of anaesthetic to help women in childbirth. But in this instance, I am referring to the 'Broad Street pump' story and the London cholera epidemic of the 1850s. An astute detector of trends in the spread of disease, Snow noticed that the people most affected by the cholera outbreak were those who used the communal water pump on Broad Street in Soho. This led him to conclude that cholera must somehow be water-borne. Failing to persuade the Westminster Council of this, he became proactive, removing the handle of the pump under cover of darkness. Obviously the authorities must have been rather slow in replacing the handle because history tells us that, before the pump became usable again, there was time for Snow to be proved correct, because the incidence of cholera among those people dropped when they were compelled to use another pump.

Like all myths (the event is true, our interpretation of it constitutes the myth), this leaves unaddressed the fact that cholera bacteria can exist in large numbers in people's intestinal tracts without them falling prey to cholera. That is, there must be another factor (or several) present to actually cause the person to develop cholera. But could it be that the presence of the cholera bacteria in the non-disease-state be more than simply neutral? Is there something to be said for the argument that, possibly, health promoters have been too simplistic in interpreting these great events in public health? That is, are we now threatening the health of our communities by being too preoccupied with cleanliness?

In an introductory chapter, one could say much more. For instance, the critical issue of HIV/AIDS has not been addressed, with all of its complex interplay of politics, big business, etc. But what has been attempted is to suggest that, not only has health promotion been with us for about as long as scientific medicine, but that it has had to be constantly flexible and responsive to its cultural context in order to be effective. Its impact is expressed in its social significance.

References

Astrow, A., Puchalski, C., Christina, M. and Sulmasy, D. (2001) 'Religion, spirituality and healthcare: social, ethical and practical considerations', *American Journal of Medicine* 110(4): 283–7.

Bellamy, D. and Pfister, D. (1992) *World Medicine*. Oxford: Blackwell.

Bentley, J. (1984) *Oberammergau: The Passion Play*. Harmondsworth: Penguin.

Defoe, D. (1966) *Journal of the Plague Year*. London: Dent.

Dubos, R. (1960) *Mirage of Health*. London: George Allen and Unwin.

Jones, W. (1945) *Hippocrates and the Corpus Hippocraticum*. Oxford: Oxford University Press.

Lalonde, M. (1974) *A New Perspective on the Health of Canadians*. Ottawa: Information Canada.

MacDonald, T. (1998) *Rethinking Health Promotion – A Global View*. London: Routledge.

MacDonald, T. (1996) 'Global Health Promotion: Challenge to a Eurocentric Concept', *British Journal of Therapy and Rehabilitation* 3(5): 279–83.

Singer, C., Underwood, C. and Underwood, E. (1962) *A Short History of Medicine*. Oxford: Clarendon Press.

Thucydides (1966) *History of the Peloponnesian War*, trans. P.A. Brunt. New English Library.

Chapter 2

The development of modern health promotion

Steven Bell

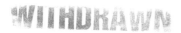

> The wheel has come full circle.
>
> (William Shakespeare, *King Lear*, Act V, Scene III)

A search of entries appearing under the subject title of 'health promotion' on the British Library website database produces a rich and varied array of publications ranging from general textbooks through policy documents to those with a specific practice-based focus. Perhaps the most interesting thing about the approximately 1,000 items that appear is, however, that none pre-date 1979.

Clearly the roots of health promotion lie in what went before. Indeed its history is as long as that of the biomedical tradition, to which it may be considered a counterpoint, and is identifiable in the deep antiquity of classical Greek and Minoan civilisations (MacDonald 1998). It is in the last 600 years or so that practice recognisable as health promotion began to take shape, and this chapter will argue that such practice was central to what was albeit a fragmented and partial approach to health prior to the Enlightenment and the dawning of modernity.

Modernity, and the genuine belief in the power of rationality for good, that is perhaps best exemplified by the Victorian obsession with progress, effectively relegated health promotion to an almost exclusively educative backwater from which it only again began to emerge in the late twentieth century. Inextricably entwined with the postmodern notions of ambiguity, subjectivity and chaos, it was really only with the *Ottawa Charter* (WHO 1986) that health promotion finally found its place increasingly in the mainstream of health policy and practice.

This chapter will relate these themes to what we today understand to be health promotion, and will conclude by considering the drivers that will shape its direction into the future.

Health in the pre-modern world

Life before the enlightenment was relatively straightforward, albeit often brutally short. The answer to the question of life, the universe and everything, while not being forty-two as suggested by Douglas Adams (1980), was just as neatly and completely explained away by the omnipotent and omniscient figure of God.

Within this context, health was a similarly simple matter, being the gift of God, and the most widespread and efficacious health intervention of the day would be the invocation of His mercy through the power of prayer. Prayer was, however, ultimately a highly pragmatic response too, for becoming sick, particularly if a surgeon was to become involved, was a risky, and expensive, business. The concept of prevention was therefore a central theme prior to the development of modern medicine, leading another Adams, on this occasion Thomas, to coin at the turn of the seventeenth century, for the first time in the English language, a rather well-known proverb:

> Prevention is so much better than the healing, because it saves the labour of being sicke.
>
> (Adams 1618: 146)

The surgeon was of course but one of three branches of medicine that existed prior to the dawn of the Enlightenment, together with the apothecary (the precursor to the pharmacist) and the physician, the latter typically tending to the needs of the more affluent. It is in the physician that a further central tenet of health promotion may be identified, the notion of holism. Andrew Boorde, a sixteenth-century physician, prescribed where to situate a house, how to organise a household, what to eat and drink and what to avoid, and what exercise to take, before moving on to more detailed methods of medical intervention (Porter 1997: 199), hinting almost 500 years in advance, at what would be Lalonde's Health Field Model (Lalonde 1974). And it didn't stop there. The holistic approach was also drawn upon heavily at the point of intervention, with morbidity being represented as an outcome of loss of balance in the vital humours. Intervention was, therefore, focused upon restoring said balance through measures, including diet, exercise and sleeping balance, as well as the application of leeches or a poultice as appropriate.

Health and modernity: the development of medicine, public health and health education

The birth of modernity is generally held to have been synonymous with that of the Enlightenment, and while no specific date exists, this watershed is usually held to have taken place around 1750. The Enlightenment was a philosophical movement stressing the importance of reason and the critical reappraisal of existing ideas and social institutions, and it brought with it two new and fundamental realities: the birth of science, and an almost unquestioning belief in progress.

Medicine, as it developed, embraced both of these, employing scientific method both to investigate and to categorise disease, and in doing so moved from a holistic model to a fundamentally biomedical and reductionist one. As a consequence, the paradigms of health promotion and medicine effectively became separate processes for the first time, with the mantle of the former being instead taken up by non-medical sections of society, with 'shortcomings in institutional medical provisions', suggests Porter (1997: 188), 'counterbalanced by the growth of writings popularising health advice'. Such educative aspects of health promotion were adopted with typical Victorian moral zeal by the church and educational systems, prompting *The Times* to assert its preference 'to take the chance of cholera and the rest than to be bullied into health' (Sutherland, 1979: 7). Improvements in housing, working practices, welfare and nursing were driven by the great eighteenth- and nineteenth-century social visionaries and reformers such as William Godwin, Robert Owen, Lord Shaftesbury, Florence Nightingale and Octavia Hill.

What was to become Public Health also emerged in a formal sense at this time, with great improvements in the condition of the overcrowded and miasmic ghettoes of many of Europe's great cities quickly making their impact felt on major sources of death and disease such as cholera, diphtheria and tuberculosis. Britain to a large extent led the way, no doubt spurred on by the 1848 cholera epidemic which claimed 60,000 lives in England and Scotland, and the influenza pandemic that killed 50,000 in London alone, with another of the great Victorian reformers, Edwin Chadwick, driving though the first Public Health Act of 1848. While it took a further 19 years to agree a Public Health Act for Scotland, other legislation at least provided for 'the removal of nuisances and the prevention of epidemic diseases' (Warren 2000: 1848) in those areas not covered by the Act. The first Public Health Medical Officers thereafter appeared in the great cities such as Glasgow, Liverpool and Birmingham during the mid-nineteenth century, and together they pioneered such developments as improved housing and sanitation, the creation of green lungs that were the great Victorian parks, and clean water supply, such as the immense scheme to supply Glasgow with water from Loch Katrine, some 50 kilometres distant.

That Chadwick was also responsible for public misery, first as assistant commissioner of the Royal Commission of Enquiry on the Poor Laws, and subsequently as the Secretary with the power to administer the Poor Law – is now a generally ignored footnote of history, other than perhaps in Ireland, where his Poor Law Amendment Act of 1834 had a knife-twisting effect on the starving years of 1845 to 1850 (Lyons 1990: 42). Ironically, however, this rather less progressive facet of Chadwick's role in social reform was also instrumental in sparking a wider public consciousness – a precursor to grassroots movements and community empowerment – with anger at the Poor Law Reform Act specifically cited as a key factor leading to the creation of the Chartist Movement of the late 1830s (Rose 1981: 259).

To compare the health education and public health movement at the time to what we understand as health promotion today, however, would be to miss perhaps the most fundamental characteristic of the latter. Interventions deriving from modernity were typified by a near paternalistic sense of duty to help the sick, the poor and the generally unfortunate, within the context of the unquestioning belief in the power for good that was science and medicine. What was lacking was any attempt to examine issues around power and control, and in this context the earlier mentioned Times editorial was essentially reasonable, albeit from a middle-class perspective of the West End, upwind and thus cocooned from the rank air of the poor quarter.

It was, however, through such work, and not through medicine, that much of the gain in health was derived through the nineteenth century. Indeed medicine, as characterised by John Knox was seen as a negative influence on this gain:

> Before 1900, doctors probably did more harm than good: between 1900 and 1930, they broke even: only since 1930, by which time the major health improvements of the present era were established, was it clear that doctors were beginning to win.
>
> (in Tones 1990: 5)

With the growth of medicine and its effectiveness, however, the public health movement went into slow decline, as science indeed began to deliver the promised land of health and prosperity. Health and prosperity were not, of course, for all, and even in wealthy Europe, significant differences remained between rich and poor. In the empires of the European nations, ironically enough, the source of much of this wealth, disease and premature death remained endemic, though through science and civilisation, such empires would, of course, deliver release for its grateful subjects.

The unshakeable belief in science as both beneficent and progressive was, however, shaken to its core by two world wars, and the capacity of science to introduce ruthless efficiency to the process of killing, culminating in its creation – through the Manhattan Project (the development of the nuclear fission bomb) – of the means to exterminate life completely.

Health and postmodernity: the age of health promotion

While associations do exist between the two constructs, postmodernity is not to be confused with postmodernism, which is essentially a literary and artistic reaction to modernism associated with the 1950s onwards. Postmodernity is instead used to capture an entire social formation and set of social and historical attitudes in what Fredric Jameson terms the 'cultural logic of late capitalism' (1984: 53). Central to this are a number of key themes, within whose mix the roots of modern health promotion are located:

1   The rise of the grassroots agenda such as the peace and women's movements in the 1950s, 1960s and 1970s, and with them the birth of community development and the concept of empowerment.
2   Cost containment concerns of the 1970s and 1980s, particularly in relation to the escalating cost of health services, culminating in the 1990s with the acknowledgement that health rationing was a reality.
3   Diminishing returns from the medical model, despite increasingly sophisticated and expensive interventions, and indeed negative returns over the last decade in areas including many of the former socialist countries and equatorial Africa, caused by a combination of social meltdown, HIV/AIDS, domestic mismanagement and international indifference.
4   The reassessment of the impact of the public health movement of the nineteenth century, and the recognition that the lessons learned still had resonance over a century later.
5   New age issues such as green concerns, with accompanying notions of equity and sustainability, formed another theme. Though perhaps of a lesser impact initially, their importance grew towards the end of the century, and were evident through the work of the WHO in respect of *Agenda 21* (United Nations 1992) and in current concerns around globalisation and economic migration.

Above all, the development of health promotion must be seen as reactive to the paradigm of the now-questioned science of progress, as ambiguity, complexity and chaos became the new reality. If modernity could be characterised as the age of science and medicine, postmodernity is the era of health promotion.

Such ambiguity and complexity is embraced by the commonly used definition of health as 'a complete state of physical, social and mental well-being, and not merely the absence of disease or disability' (WHO 1948: 100), a definition fundamental for its rediscovery of holism, and also for characterising health as a state of being, which is therefore brought about by a creative and positive act.

Though the World Health Organization is unquestionably key to the development of modern health promotion, the first true framework for such positive actions was proposed in 1974 by Marc Lalonde, then Minister for Health in Canada, in *A New Perspective on the Health of Canadians* (Lalonde 1974). The Health Field Model developed therein, with its headings of environment, lifestyles, healthcare organisations and human biology, placed Canada at the forefront of driving the new paradigm for over a decade. In anticipating by a quarter of a century, for instance, the three action levels of 'Life Circumstances', 'Lifestyle' and 'Health Topics'

(Scottish Office 1999: 7) that would come to shape British health strategy, its importance in underpinning our understanding of health and its determinants to this day cannot be understated.

Many existing health promotion texts deal with the role of Marc Lalonde rather dismissively as a side-issue. Indeed, some do not mention him at all. Yet the modern development of health promotion is directly traceable to the Lalonde Report, as *A New Perspective on the Health of Canadians* has come to be known. It was written at a time when various commentators on the Canadian health scene were making observations to the effect that increasing the amount of money spent by government on healthcare was no longer having an impact on actual health indices.

Lalonde's argument was that a great increase in the impact of health spending could be brought about by empowering everyone in the community to identify their health agenda, and to develop agencies by which these could be 'advocated' at the neighbourhood level, and then mediated through open access to government agencies. A particularly fine discussion of the issues raised by Lalonde, in which due credit is given to the importance of his ideas to the development of current thinking, is contained in the pointedly titled *Why Are Some People Healthy and Others Not?* (Evans et al. 1995), in particular in Chapter 2, 'Producing Health, Consuming Health Care'.

Aeron Antonovsky further developed this idea in the context of his salutogenic model of health, which embraced the notion of empowerment in his Sense of Coherence (SOC) construct. Antonovsky's studies caused him to consider what it was about survivors of horrors such as the Holocaust that distinguished them from the majority who succumbed, and led him to contend that 'strengthening the SOC of people would be a major contributor of their move towards health' (1996: 16). Empowerment is therefore characterised as more than merely a process, but as an end in itself. This contrasts sharply with the often confused concept of consumerism, which is essentially an individual and economic construct, compared with the collective and social construct of empowerment. The term 'salutogenic', it should be noted, derives from the Greek salus, meaning health, and genesis, meaning birth.

This new understanding, particularly in the failure of medicine to address the huge differences in health that existed both within, and between countries, led to the development of the 'WHO Health For All by the Year 2000' movement. This can be best described as a crusade-like call for all governments of the world to make Health For All their central priority for the remainder of the century. It was signed in 1977 at the thirteenth WHO Congress, at Alma-Ata in the former Soviet Union. Alma-Ata, as many students of nursing will know, resonates with historical allusions to the abuse of health. It is only a few miles from Scutari, the location of the notorious military field hospital at which Florence Nightingale nursed injured soldiers in appalling conditions during the Crimean War (1853–6). A most vibrant account of this unfortunate episode in our health history can be found in Cecil Woodham-Smith's book, Florence Nightingale (1820–1910).

The WHO Congress established thirty-eight objectives for health, based upon ensuring the great prerequisites of education, shelter, clean water, sanitation and freedom from poverty and war (WHO 1977). Perhaps unsurprisingly, the relevance of the declaration and its impact was felt largely in developing countries, as the developed world, no doubt smug in its self-perceived success in delivering the prerequisites for health, did little.

In addition, for a Western government to assume an interventionist approach to addressing health abuses arising directly from their own capitalist social policies, would constitute a contradiction; indeed, it would be an anathema to the new right-wing administrations so characteristic of the individualist 1980s, both in Europe and the USA. In making this observation, reference is explicitly made to the administrations of Prime Minister Margaret Thatcher in Britain, and President Ronald Reagan in the USA.

Famously, and illustrating its discomfort with the issue, the Thatcher government tried to suppress the publication of the Black Report on *Inequalities in Health* (Townsend and Davidson 1982), by arranging its release on a bank holiday.

The Ottawa Charter

For health promotion, the newly emerging discipline of the 1980s, the World Health Organization and Canada would again provide the impetus through the *Ottawa Charter on Health Promotion* (WHO 1986). Fundamental for reinforcing the issue of empowerment in respect of health, the *Ottawa Charter* defined health promotion as 'the process of enabling people to take control over, and to improve their health', and identified five key levers which health promotion should employ:

* building healthy public policy;
* creating supporting environments;
* strengthening community action;
* developing personal skills and capacities;
* reorienting health services.

Crucially, the *Ottawa Charter* was also closely linked to the launch of the Healthy Cities Movement by the European Office of the World Health Organization in 1986. This was a mechanism for circumventing less than supportive national governments, by implementing Health For All at a sub-national level. Recognising the fact that the majority of the world's population would live in cities by the year 2000, the movement followed closely in the tradition of the public medical officers of a century earlier by focusing on the city as an entity, though now as a dynamic and living organism whose every system has profound implications for health. In this sense, Healthy Cities was 'marking the point at which the Health For All Strategy was "taken off the shelves and put into the streets" ' (Ashton and Seymour 1988: 154).

The development of Healthy Cities also marked the emergence of the settings approach (Downie *et al.* 1996: 63) which would have significant impact on the organisation and delivery of health promotion at a functional level. At its most holistic level, this approach shifts the balance away from health promotion merely happening in a given setting, to generating settings that were also inherently health-promoting in their own right. Examples of such approaches include the development of health-promoting hospitals as a mechanism, first proposed by the World Health Organization (WHO 1991), for truly reorienting health services, and health-promoting schools (WHO, Council of Europe and Commission of the European Community 1993).

In countries such as Britain, the 1990s saw an increasing interest and investment in the role of health promotion, though principally at the local level, with more of an educative emphasis being placed at a national level within the context of the individualist and consumerist philosophy of the then Conservative administration. The election in 1997 of the New Labour government in Britain brought a seismic shift, with health promotion and public health being mainstreamed at the heart of government policy, to the extent that one would indeed be forgiven for believing that health promotion was a new big idea. As we have seen, the discovery by the New Labour government of life circumstances, lifestyle and health topics as the theatres in which health improvement will be played out owes more to history than it did to inspiration; therefore it is fair to consider New Labour, and not its policy direction, to be the big idea.

Whether or not the shift is complete, however, is a moot point, as the confusion referred to earlier between empowerment and consumerism remains an issue, with references to health education and personal responsibility still commonplace. In saying this, however, I do not intend to suggest discontent, as there is indeed an important role for health promotion in attempts to increase the appropriate use of health services and promote health citizenship. The point is merely made to highlight that such a perspective is but a superficial reflection of what health promotion can bring to an integrated and multidisciplinary approach to public health.

Health improvement in the twenty-first century

Perhaps the best example of this increasing integration can be seen in Scotland within the context of the review and development of public health (see Chapter 12). At the inception of this process in 1999, it was explicitly acknowledged that the broad view of public health adopted 'derives from the international health promotion work underway since the mid 1970s and the proposal of the World Health Organization for "Health for all by the

Year 2000"' (Scottish Executive 1999: 21). Driven forward by Professor Phil Hanlon, Director of the Public Health Institute for Scotland (PHIS), whose credentials included being a former Director of Health Promotion for Greater Glasgow Health Board and lecturing in Health Promotion at the University of Glasgow, the development of NHS Boards as public health organisations explicitly emphasises the importance of the *Ottawa Charter*. Somewhat pointedly, however, the reference to this seminal instrument omits the important and qualifying suffix of 'for health promotion' (PHIS 2002: 11).

This omission is worryingly characteristic of current developments, where health promotion is regarded almost as an afterthought, and the widespread assumption exists that the use of inclusive and health-promotion-reflective language is enactive of change itself. The weaknesses of health promotion in relation to its medical and nursing partners leaves a concern that, following the mainstreaming of the health promotion philosophy, the latter groups have re-emerged to claim the tradition and territory as their own, with the subsequent lessening and even sidelining of the role of health promotion specialists. It remains to be seen what distinctiveness and influence remain for health promotion if and when the proposals for a unified and single collegiate structure for the public health workforce are implemented.

In a similar vein, the interchangeable employment of the terms 'public health' and 'health improvement' is a regrettable development, especially where the latter term has been adopted as a functional description. Free from the baggage of politics or alignment with a specific functional or occupational grouping, health improvement had the opportunity of becoming an umbrella term defining the collective mission of all of those working towards the improvement of health, including those in public health medicine, dentistry and nursing, and health promotion, as well as those from housing, environmental health, and the myriad others engaged within a multidisciplinary public health workforce.

It should be stated that both the increased emphasis on health improvement and the drive towards integration are very welcome trends, though the fear must remain that retrenchment following a change in national political leadership may return the agenda to a much narrower one: we must not forget the lessons of history in the 1980s. The key difference, however, is that there will not necessarily be the bulwark of a distinctive health promotion movement acting as champion for the social science and salutogenic perspective.

And so with the wheel come full circle, and the counterpoint traditions of Hygeia and Panacea, of health promotion and medicine, essentially aligned for the first time since the dawn of the Enlightenment, or even, arguably, for over 3,000 years (MacDonald 1998: 7), we must be on our guard that health promotion does not become subsumed and even lost as a distinctive though complementary melody. For if it is, the lesson of history is that health promotion would simply have to be reinvented.

References

Adams, D. (1980) *The Hitchhiker's Guide to the Galaxy*. London: Pan Books.

Adams, T. (1618) 'Happiness of Church', in J. Simpson (1981) *The Concise Oxford Dictionary of Proverbs*, Oxford: Oxford University Press.

Antonovsky, A. (1996) 'The Salutogenic Model as a Theory to Guide Health Promotion', *Health Promotion International* 11(1): 11–18.

Ashton, J. and Seymour, H. (1988) *The New Public Health*. Milton Keynes: Open University Press.

Downie, R.S., Tannahill, C. and Tannahill A. (1996) *Health Promotion Models and Values,* 2nd edn. Oxford: Oxford University Press.

Evans, R.G., Barer, M.L. and Marmor, T.R. (1995) *Why Are Some People Healthy and Others Not? The Determinants of the Health of Population*. New York: Aldine De Gruyter.

Jameson, F. (1984) 'Postmodernism, or the Cultural Logic of Late Capitalism', *New Left Review* 146: 53–92.

Lalonde, M. (1974) *A New Perspective on the Health of Canadians*. Ottawa: Information Canada.

Lyons, F.S.L. (1990) *Ireland Since the Famine*. London: Fontana.

MacDonald, T. (1999) *Rethinking Health Promotion: A Global Approach*. London: Routledge.

PHIS (Public Health Institute for Scotland) (2002) *NHS Boards as Public Health Organisations: A Report from the Scottish Directors of Public Health Group and the Public Health Institute for Scotland*. Glasgow: PHIS.

Porter, R. (1997) *The Greatest Benefit to Mankind: A Medical History of Humanity from Antiquity to the Present*. London: Fontana.

Rose, M.E. (1981) 'Social Change and the Industrial Revolution', in R. Floud and D. McCloskey (eds) *The Economic History of Britain Since 1700, Vol. 1: 1700–1860*. Cambridge: Cambridge University Press.

Scottish Executive (1999) *Review of the Public Health Function in Scotland*. Edinburgh: Scottish Executive.

Scottish Office (1999) *Towards a Healthier Scotland* Edinburgh: The Stationery Office.

Sutherland, I. (1979) *Health Education: Perspectives and Choice*. London: Allen and Unwin.

Tones, B.K. (1990) *The Power to Choose: Health Education and the New Public Health*. Health Education Unit, Leeds Polytechnic.

Townsend, P. and Davidson, N. (1982) *Inequalities in Health: The Black Report*. Harmondsworth: Penguin.

United Nations (1992) *Agenda 21, as adopted by the United Nations Conference on the Environment and Development (UNCED), Rio de Janeiro, Brazil*. New York: United Nations Division for Sustainable Development.

Warren, M.D. (2000) *A Chronology of State Medicine, Public Health, Welfare and Related Services in Britain 1066–1999*. London: Faculty of Public Health Medicine.

WHO (World Health Organization) (1948) 'Preamble to the Constitution of the World Health Organization as adopted by the International Health Conference, New York, 19–22 June 1946; signed on 22 July 1946 by the representatives of 61 States', *Official Records of the World Health Organization* 2.

WHO (World Health Organization) (1977) *Alma-Ata Declaration*. Geneva: WHO.

WHO (World Health Organization) (1986) *Ottawa Charter for Health Promotion*. Geneva: WHO.

WHO (World Health Organization) (1991) *The Budapest Declaration on Health Promoting Hospitals – WHO Business Meeting, Healthy Hospitals – Next Steps on the Way to the Health Promoting Hosptial* (Budapest, Hungary, 31 May–1 June 1991), Geneva: WHO.

WHO (World Health Organization), Council of Europe and Commission of the European Communities (1993) *The European Network of Health Promoting Schools*. Copenhagen: WHO.

Woodham-Smith, C. (1991) *The Reason Why*. Harmondsworth: Penguin.

Chapter 3

The idea of 'participation' in health research and evaluation

Conan Leavey

Introduction

This chapter draws on our experience of teaching and working with participatory health research and evaluation methodologies. At a very basic level the impetus for writing this chapter emerged from a number of conversations I had with colleagues about what we perceived to be an emerging orthodoxy concerning 'participation' in health research and evaluation. For the most part, we were positive about these ideas. We discussed them with graduate and postgraduate students working in health promotion and used them in our work as researchers and consultants. However, I was also uncomfortable with how some of these principles seemed to work in practice. As a response, I have set out to clarify my concerns for the way in which 'participation' is currently conceived and practised, focusing on a number of organising principles which are currently popular. My conclusions do not necessarily represent the views of my colleagues and while I feel that the idea of participation has a lot to offer, I will present two sets of qualifying arguments: first, that participation does not automatically make for better research and evaluation – it is only as useful as the context and practitioner permits, given their understanding of and commitment to the methodology; second, that deeper systemic problems exist whereby currently fashionable epistemological arguments can circumvent legitimate concerns about 'bias' in health research and evaluation projects.

The idea of participation

The purpose of this section is to identify the emergence of the idea of 'participation' in health research and evaluation. At the outset I would like to make it clear that health evaluation is increasingly regarded as a discipline in its own right, with its own philosophy and methodological tool kit. I am presently unpersuaded by these arguments. To the extent that health evaluators share the methods and philosophical concerns of other social scientists, I see every reason to locate evaluation firmly in the applied branch of the social sciences, that is, one that assesses and informs planned interventions in health in accordance with the best principles of social science practice.

The concept of 'participation' has its origins in the wider social sciences, where ideas about the need for solution-focused and inclusive approaches to knowledge-generation have emerged as key philosophical and methodological principles in disciplines as diverse as social psychology, organisational science, educational theory, whole-systems thinking and complexity science (Hart and Bond 1995; Stringer 1996; Greenwood and Levin 1998). These disciplines have fed into the idea that social science research would benefit from being less expert-led and should incorporate people more democratically into the design, collection and analysis of the data.

The impetus behind this development has combined two closely linked sets of ideas. The first set of ideas argues that social science research is more likely to produce effective solutions to social problems if it acknowledges that people are 'experts' on their own situation and can work towards their own solutions. This will also contribute towards a fairer society by including the views, aspirations and life experiences of groups of people who are normally excluded from the planning and decision-making processes. The second set of ideas argues that conventional social research has been limited by a nineteenth-century view of what constitutes 'good' science. This has denigrated non-scientific ways of knowing the world, led to a mechanical view of human agency and generally produced research which ignores people's 'humanness' (Lincoln and Guba 1985: 27). I want to suggest that the first set of ideas concerns itself with the political ramifications of how social science is organised and practised in society, rather than with its fundamental intellectual premises; the second set of ideas promotes a non-positivist view of science and suggests an alternative epistemology for the study of social life.

The emergence of solution-focused and participatory approaches to social research is usually accredited to Kurt Lewin and his colleagues, in the USA, and the Tavistock Institute for Human Relations, in Britain, although this analysis ignores the development of these ideas in the Third World (Holter and Schwartz-Barcott 1993). Lewin trained in social and experimental psychology and developed a quasi-experimental approach to solving social and technical problems in post-war Europe and America. His research papers cover an extraordinary range of topics, including encouraging housewives to cook tripe, preparing Jewish children to cope with discrimination, and resolving face-to-face conflict in marriage, among factory workers and between minority groups.

Contemporary practitioners might balk at his reference to 'social engineering' and his idea of 'participation' now appears rather limited. However, the ideas of Lewin and his colleagues have been extremely influential in the Norwegian Industrial Democracy Project and in educational theory, where they have been translated into concerns about optimising people's learning experiences. Lewin was committed to the idea that research itself should create change and stated that 'research that produces nothing but books will not suffice' (Lewin 1948: 203). Working on the principle that the best way to understand something is to try and change it, he pioneered a model of research in which action, research and training formed a triangle 'that should be kept together for the sake of any of its corners' (Lewin 1948: 206). He imagined research to 'proceed in a spiral of steps each of which is composed of a circle of planning, action, and fact finding about the result of that action'. This approach anticipated ideas in both education and organisational theory about the importance of 'active' rather than 'passive' learning. The importance of constant cycles of action and reflection in knowledge acquisition underwrite most participatory approaches today (Greenwood and Levin 1998).

Whole-systems thinking (Capra 1996), complexity theory (Dean 1997), chaos theory and quantum physics (Zohar 1991; Zohar and Marshall 1993) have also been used to support the idea that the researcher and researched are intimately bound together in the process of knowledge-generation. They have furnished social science with a 'scientific' epistemology that tries to escape the constraints of the positivist world-view. These perspectives apply insights from the biological and physical sciences to an understanding of how organisations and socio-cultural systems operate. They rely on a holistic view of the world, where social phenomena and biological phenomena are thought to share the same qualities as 'systems'. Social phenomena are perceived to be the outcome of dynamic interactions between individuals, the social systems in which they operate and a wider ecology of systems interacting to form macro-systems.

During the 1990s, complexity science and whole-systems thinking provided an intellectual backdrop to the King's Fund initiatives to stimulate innovation in primary care (Thomas 2002). It emphasised a multi-pronged approach to changing organisations and promoted the idea that the researcher is a dynamic part of the system being 'studied', rather than an independent observer.

This eclectic intellectual genealogy underscores a variety of research traditions that are currently gaining in popularity, such as action research, participatory research, participatory action research and collaborative inquiry (Whyte 1991). The resulting confusion has been called 'terminological anarchism', where the conceptual boundaries between different strands are often unclear (Kalleberg 1990). While any attempt to establish definitions will not be exhaustive, I argue that the concept of participation in health research and evaluation is closely associated with other concerns, as follows:

1 the development of an anti-positivist epistemology suited to the diverse experience of health and illness in society;
2 the desire to solve 'real'-world problems rather than produce 'academic knowledge' or 'knowledge for its own sake';
3 a concern with social justice and the empowerment of excluded groups;

4   the need to create learning organisations that respond effectively to the health needs of different communities.

Taken together these form the backbone of participatory approaches to health research and evaluation.

Anti-positivism

There is a strong vein of anti-positivism in participatory approaches, stemming from a widespread disillusionment in some quarters of the social science community with the appropriateness of conventional theory and methods to the study of human groups and organisations (Lincoln and Guba 1985; Whyte 1991; Reason 1988; Hart and Bond 1995). There is a feeling that social scientists have been unduly influenced by nineteenth-century notions drawn from the natural sciences – such as laboratory-type experimentation, the search for immutable social facts and the invariant laws governing social life. It is argued that these are neither ethical nor accurate ways of understanding the social world.

Schutz (1954) neatly pointed out that social scientists are different from natural scientists because they have a *reflective* subject matter – other thinking, feeling, human beings who will construct meanings, hold values and have a dynamic relationship with those studying them. The Hawthorne Effect, for instance, was coined to describe the phenomenon that whenever special attention is paid to a group of people, their behaviour changes simply as a consequence of being observed (Gregory 1987). Even in the more 'naturally occurring' investigations typical of ethnography, people's behaviour will be influenced by the researcher's degree of interaction and relative social position to the group (Fay 1996). While 'objectivity' may work for the exploration of natural phenomena, the argument goes, it does not work for people operating in complex and dynamic situations. The factors influencing people's decisions and actions are too fluid to yield invariant laws of behaviour. The prejudices and motives of researchers interweave with those of their subjects, so that social scientists feel that 'interpretations' rather than 'facts' should be the aim of their research. In short, the methodological monism of John Stuart Mill – who argued that the aims of the natural and social sciences should be identical – is a chimera that renders the practice of social science virtually impossible.

These anti-positivist challenges come in 'soft' and 'hard' forms. The soft version suggests that *all* systems of knowledge-production (including science) are value-laden; the selection of research topics, and the gathering and interpretation of scientific data are shaped by professional ambitions, practical constraints, and ideological and political hegemonies (Greenwood and Levin 1998: 57–64). This does not mean that objective knowledge is impossible, but that historical and cultural lenses filter what researchers think is important and how they subsequently interpret their findings. The hard version argues that objective knowledge of the world *in toto* is impossible, not just because of personal and ideological bias, but because all human processes of perception influence the world they perceive, right down to the sub-atomic level. Lessons are drawn from Heisenberg's Uncertainty Principle and the conundrum of Schrödinger's Cat, wherein it is suggested that a physicist interferes with sub-atomic articles by the very act of measuring them. Hermeneutics, postmodernism and phenomenology are combined with these observations from quantum physics to lend the weight to the idea put forward by social scientists that the processes of human observation are indivisible from the processes of social life (Fay 1996).

What impact has this general anti-positivism had on the social sciences and on health research and evaluation? In its weak version, these arguments have led to a certain degree of methodological relativism which rejects the idea that any given set of research methods can be 'objective' in the sense that they stand aside from human value systems. It has encouraged researchers to be more critical of whose interests their research findings serve and to deconstruct the complex web of presuppositions they hold by virtue of their gender, sexuality, class or ethnicity. It is now standard practice for undergraduate students to examine how their expectations and prejudices may have influenced their interpretation of the empirical data and to support their interpretations with reference to a range of diffuse 'quality' concepts. Consequently, there has been a move away from expert-led models of inquiry, where researchers are seen as having privileged access to knowledge and where mathematical data is seen as *prima facie* evidence for the objectivity of their conclusions (Jayaratne 1993) towards approaches which explore 'insider' or emic views of complex health problems and health-related behaviours. Greater respect is accorded to 'non-scientific' ways of knowing the world, and more interest is shown in how individuals and groups of individuals construe the world and their place within it. Everyone is now assumed to be an expert on his or her own life-circumstances and experiences.

At the rhetorical level at least, the views of non-professionals, lay experts and the insights of local knowledge are accorded equal status with the views of academics, professionals and research experts. This has resulted in a rise in the acceptability of qualitative methods, as researchers have picked up on the methods that convincingly convey the life-world of respondents. Interviews and focus groups have moved out of the shadows, where they were seen as a 'soft' complement to 'hard' quantitative data, to take a prominent role in health research and evaluation. More than before, researchers are using qualitative methods to ask people about their health needs, or their experiences of services, or the impact of health interventions, on behalf of those who shape policy and prioritise services. The move has been away from imposing expert frameworks on people, towards a greater humility in the practice of social science research.

In its 'hard' version, anti-positivism has led to a more radical critique of social science practice. Sokal and Bricmont (1998) have called this critique 'epistemological relativism' and it has an anti-science flavour. In these arguments, science is criticised not only for the way it is organised and practised in society (for example, it serves the interest of capitalist economics, it has been used to support racist and sexist ideologies, etc.) but at an axiomatic level for being inherently anti-human, anti-nature, patriarchal, linear, or in some other way incommensurate with the full flourishing of human potential. It has led to a climate in which personal and group subjectivities are valued above all else, and where suspicion falls on researchers who provide explanations that fall outside the 'insider's' frame of reference. I will later return to how this shift from methodological to epistemological relativism may be problematic for health research and evaluation.

Inclusive approaches to research

Parallel with the growth of non-positivist epistemologies has been an increasing acceptance of more inclusive or participatory approaches to research. What is meant by these terms tends to vary but, broadly speaking, they indicate an attempt to democratise the research process by turning people from 'subjects' to 'participants' in that research process. There is no consensus over the nature or extent of participation needed in the research process – it varies according to the nature of the problem and the philosophical commitments of those initiating the research. Industrial management has favoured a cautious definition where some of the people participate in the stages of the research process in order to improve conditions for workers and increase productivity (Whyte 1991). In the Third World, 'participation' has stressed the radicalising dimension, in which the researcher moves people towards their needs and aspirations (Rahman 1993). In management and organisational development, all the participants in a research project are expected to become co-researchers, promoting a model which combines elements of organisational change, professional development and personal growth (Reason 1988).

The new orthodoxy is that more can be achieved when research is done *with* people rather than *to* people (Reason 1988). There appears to be both a utilitarian and ethical imperative behind this development. First, there is the failure of conventional science to solve pressing social problems combined with a growing scepticism towards the perceived benefits of science, medicine and technology (Norgaard 1994). Second, there often prevails an expressly political concern that marginalised groups should be involved in the research process. The representation of excluded people and the articulation of the 'view from below' (Mies 1993) has become an explicit value-base for social constructionism (Berger and Luckmann 1966; Stainton Rogers 1991), naturalistic inquiry (Lincoln and Guba 1985), interpretivism (Schwandt 1994), feminist and standpoint epistemologies (Denzin 1997).

There is evidence that participatory methodologies can produce practical solutions and develop useful theory. They have been used to address problems of productivity in post-war Europe (Lewin 1946), worker/management relations in industry during the 1970s and 1980s (Whyte 1991), and major processes of socio-technological change by encouraging fuller hands-on decision-making from workers (Greenwood and Levin 1998). The Third World approach has focused on community participation from marginalised groups in identifying health needs, devising and evaluating health programmes (Tandon 1993; de Koning and Martin 1996). Community involvement and respecting local people's knowledge has proven integral to rural health development projects (Gardner and Lewis 1996), the international primary care movement and alternative development models which seek to increase political and economic participation through education (Freire 1970; Rahman 1993; Munck and O'Hearn 1999). The concept of participation has become a nearly universal part of development philosophy (Cooke and Kothari, 2001).

In Western Europe, the idea of participation has taken two overlapping forms. In the first, community participation has become a central tenet of the health promotion movement. Community development projects have helped to reveal how poverty and poor health are caused by social and economic structures based on class and power, rather than individual failings. Later community development work in health promotion has focused on helping community groups to address their own health issues and has highlighted the problems faced by Western industrialised countries when restructuring power relations in the interests of marginalised or low-status groups (Hart and Bond 1995).

The second form of participation has focused on improving the delivery of services for marginalised groups by changing health and welfare organisations, rather than getting communities to directly address their own problems (Carr and Kemmis 1986). This type of research has employed a 'professionalising' and less radical form of participation that has concentrated on helping practitioners to improve services and practice on behalf of the users (Hart and Bond 1995: 40). The aim is to investigate the problems identified by professionals and improve practice over time by developing a prudent understanding of what should be done in practical situations. It is appropriate whenever 'specific knowledge is required for a specific problem in a specific situation' (Cohen and Manion 1984: 48). It focuses on the interaction of the researcher with the professionals, who are approached as experts on the workplace under study because they know the setting 'from the inside' (Holter and Schwartz-Barcott 1993).

When marginalised groups have been involved in this process, it is often with the aim of increasing their participation in health promotion services. The involvement of users may vary depending on the commitment of the researcher and practitioners. Macaulay *et al.* (1999) argue that high levels of community and lay involvement help practitioners design research protocols suited to improving services in line with community needs. Other researchers regard the relationship between the practitioners and the researcher as central, and the researcher's task is to facilitate a discussion of underlying problems on a personal as well as an organisational level (Holter and Schwartz-Barcott 1993).

In formal healthcare settings, the participation of professionals has been used to catalyse the research process and generate the levels of commitment needed for organisational change in bureaucratic structures (Hart and Bond 1995). It hands over the agenda-setting to practitioners who are close to problems grounded in daily experience. Involvement in the research process increases the acceptability of the project to the research community, commitment to the findings and the likelihood that these findings will be used to initiate another project or extended to another setting. Winter (1989) has argued that individual reports of participatory research can inform other health professionals of critical issues relevant to improving services more generally. Comparative descriptions of other people's practice can be used to reflect critically on one's own working practice and prompt further action for improvement (Bloor and McKeganey 1989).

The most striking difference between these different types of participation and conventional social science research has been the democratisation of the research process. Conventional models of research treat members of communities or organisations as passive subjects, with some of them participating only to the extent of agreeing to a research project, producing data and receiving the results. Applied research has been a notable exception to this model but it still 'professional-expert' to the extent that it is the researcher who designs the project, gathers the data, interprets the findings and delivers the recommendations (Whyte 1991). In contrast, participatory approaches involve the organisation or community under study actively involving itself throughout the research process, from the initial design of the project to the presentation of the results and the discussion of their implications for action (Reason 1988; Elden and Levin 1991).

This approach fits with non-positivist ideas about the co-generative nature of knowledge production in the social sciences. Participatory approaches are not expected to produce 'value-free' information. Research-ers are expected to examine their own values and the partisan aims of their stakeholders during the research process (Stringer 1996). It is assumed that people can generate knowledge as part of a systematic inquiry process based on their own categories and frameworks. These interpretive frameworks are augmented by, rather than rely on, the researcher's own interpretation of the findings, creating a third interpretive framework. This framework becomes part of the data and the basis for collective learning through cycles of involvement and reflection. It is an approach that aims to create a learning environment in which the research community produces findings of local relevance and effective ideas can be diffused to different contexts or settings (Greenwood and Levin 1998).

Current trends

I briefly want to examine why the idea of 'participation' in health research and evaluation has become so prevalent. First, it fits in with the holistic definition of 'health' currently popular in health promotion. Health promotion has moved on from measuring health outcomes in narrowly defined medical terms towards a multi-dimensional concept that embraces notions of wellness, wholeness and a variety of individual and group subjectivities. This has encouraged researchers to use a range of qualitative and participatory methods to reflect the diversity of health and illness experiences in society. Lincoln (1990) argues that it is this straightforward observational and inter-view data, rather than participation *per se*, that can help us to understand the socially determined nature of health behaviour on which grounded theories of human health can be built. The articulation of minority group voices, whether to express the experiences of racism, poverty, sexism, living with a chronic condition, or the articulation of cultural health beliefs or dissatisfaction with services, are best accessed using qualitative research methods. This 'down-ward' focus has led researchers to be more sensitive to their personal and disciplinary prejudices while making a concentrated effort to understand the group and individual subjectivities of others' experience.

Second, the idea of democratising the research process fits well with other ideas about how our public and personal lives can be improved. The right to 'participation' has become a guiding trope for our society, codified by an increasing web of surveys, focus groups and consumer representation groups in which we are asked for, and expected to provide, feedback on a range of issues or products. The idea of participation has become a political impera-tive for reforming our public services, through more client participation, more intersectoral collaboration, more joined-up thinking.

There has been an opportunity here for both the 'professionalising' and 'radical' types of participatory researcher (Springett and Leavey 1995). The more expressly political have worked with community groups to identify health needs and mobilise 'social capital' to improve conditions. The 'professional-ising' types have worked with organisations to improve health services in line with individuals' and communities' needs. Managers and clinicians in primary care groups are increasingly expected to engage in collaborative projects with the public, assess health needs, reduce health inequalities, listen to users' views, work in partnership with local agencies and to be able to use research findings to improve services. In primary care, quality assurance is provided by agencies such as the National Institute of Clinical Excellence and the Commission for Health Improvements, on the one hand, and significant elements of peer review and public scrutiny through user involvement, on the other hand. Fisher *et al.* (1999) observe that few general practices have prior experience of involving patients in practice decision-making, and that the government has provided little conceptual or managerial guidance on public involvement. It is unsurprising, therefore, that participatory approaches appear well placed to help health professionals meet these top-down and bottom-up agendas because they provide flexible models which combine the expertise of both local people and health professionals (Oldham and Rutter 1999: 748).

National programmes, such as the Health Action Zones, Health Improvement Schemes and Healthy Living Centres, have reached a stage at which they now require systematic evaluation. It is argued that participatory researchers have an opportunity to feed up the view from the ground-level on how guiding principles such as equity, partnership working, community inclusion and whole-systems thinking have been put into practice.

Problems with the idea of participation

In this section, I will raise a number of concerns about the way in which the idea of participation manifests itself in health research and evaluation. The first concern is about the gap between rhetoric and reality. Cooke and Kothari (2001) refer to a disturbing disjuncture between the almost universally fashionable rhetoric of participation on the one hand, with its promises of empowerment and inclusivity, and what actually happens when consultants practise participatory approaches, on the other. I have already noted that participation can take more or less radical forms depending on the context of the research and the methodological commitment of the researcher. Now that the concept of participation has moved into establishment thinking, there is a risk that it will be increasingly de-radicalised to fit the diverse contexts in which it is expected to operate. There is a real danger that participation, in spite of the well-meant intentions of its proponents, can lead to a tokenistic representation that is self-defeating. The current vogue for short-term user-involvement groups, where lay representatives and service providers are brought together in collaborative forums, can lead to unrealistic expectations if participants do not adequately appreciate the structural constraints operating on health professionals. Consultation with marginalised groups does not magically lead to improvement in services unless combined with a genuine political will to do so, and many researchers wonder privately to what extent their services are required so that the criteria for 'participation' have at least been met on paper.

One must also consider to what extent participation has become a buzzword that oils the wheels of academia. Like a drawing by Escher, where water miraculously flows through a series of down hill channels only to become its own source, the idea of participation flows from policy level to ground level and back again. When researchers are hired as consultants to evaluate the success of health interventions or community projects, their methods frequently focus on gathering the perceptions and experiences of co-ordinators and community groups competing in a fierce 'bidding culture' with access to limited supplies of funding (Dunmore 2002). Participatory evaluators join the loop when they use qualitative methods to evaluate projects in which the participants' own utterances become the evidence to support their success. Under these conditions, there is considerable pressure on people to give a positive spin to what they do, and it is difficult to see where any radical critiques of the system can emerge. In a recent study, co-ordinators reported that they used terms like 'social capital' and 'social inclusion' because they appeared in official documents, not because they necessarily understood the terms or felt they adequately described grass-roots projects (Chendo 2002).

'Local knowledge' and 'community' take on a strange quality when community groups accrete around funding opportunities and local knowledge is groomed to fit the criteria set by national evaluative frameworks. Mosse (2001: 19) refers to the 'rather peculiar type of knowledge' produced by participatory events that take place in the presence of local authority officers or outsiders. In such circumstances, participatory methods are likely to produce 'planning knowledge', in which community groups and co-ordinators collude in a kind of mutually beneficial knowledge, oriented 'upwards' to justify higher policy goals. Community groups are required to demonstrate their efficacy in terms of vaguely operationalised notions of social capital and empowerment, part of a specialised vocabulary that community spokespeople must master in verbal and written form to produce the proposals necessary to secure further funding. I want to suggest that the idea of 'community' is gradually being removed from the experiences of ordinary people, rationalised by bureaucratic structures and professional academics, where it re-enters the consciousness of the population in the form of reified and selective notions of what a community is and what it should do for people. This amounts to community 'invention' rather than community 'participation' and the majority of planners and consultants are part of the process because their broadly leftist/liberal sensibilities will ensure that some well-organised grassroots movements will not make it on to the community development agenda.

The idea that participants should decide the aims, outcomes and methods for research starts to look very different depending on whether it is done with the powerless or the powerful. How are researchers to avoid getting locked into webs of patronage when they are hired by organisations to evaluate health and community interventions positioned in a bidding culture?

Part of the problem seems to be the canonisation of the idea of participation at the philosophical level. The assumption that participatory research is always better research ignores the fact that researchers are frequently hired by organisations and government departments to provide evidence that validates their goals and outcomes. I want to suggest that references by social scientists to chaos theory, quantum theory and holistic science tend to support the view that the universe is essentially unknowable because it is bound to human perception, and that the researcher and the researched are epistemologically inseparable. This is no less problematic than the counter-claim that social scientists stand outside the social world and can arrive at ultimate objective truths about it. The second set of arguments denies the politically loaded nature of social knowledge, the first set writes it off as unavoidable and inevitable. Both arguments legitimate a position in which social scientists are near-sighted with respect to the influences of power and politics on knowledge production.

Two scientists, Alan Sokal and Jean Bricmont, became infamous for duping the social science community in 1996 with a spoof paper called 'Transgressing the Boundaries: Toward a Transformative Hermeneutics of Quantum Gravity'. The paper was accepted and published to considerable critical acclaim by the American cultural-studies journal, *Social Text*, despite the fact that it 'is brimming with absurdities and blatant non-sequiturs' (Sokal and Bricmont 1998: 1). They perpetrated the hoax as a statement against what they saw as a growing 'radical relativism' among social scientists that regarded modern science as nothing more than a 'myth', a 'narration' or a 'social construction'. They argue against the idea that scientific terms and concepts have immediate and deep implications for the study of society, and point out that 'throwing around' references to quantum and chaos theories serves only to mystify the social sciences with erudition taken wildly out of context (1998: x). In truth, most of us would be uneasy if quantum or chaos theories became the guiding principles behind the legal process, investigative journalism, auto-mobile repairs or any other system of knowledge that impacts directly on people's welfare.

Finally, I want to suggest that references to the new physics, whole-systems thinking and holistic science – as a rationale for why 'participation' makes for better research – repeats the methodological monism of John Stuart Mill in a different form; that is, it indicates to social scientists that they should look to the natural sciences for their guiding principles and philosophy. I think this is a mistake and we need a much more humanistic and politically savvy version of when 'participation' is appropriate or useful. The political impetus behind the idea of participation – to give a voice to the voiceless – is in danger of being replaced by a sophistry that lets the powerful sing to a tune of their own making. Health research and evaluation that is participatory is not necessarily better than other forms of research. It depends on how it is done, and with whom.

References

Berger, P. and Luckmann, T. (1966) *The Social Construction of Reality*. London: Allan Lane.

Bloor, M. and McKegnay, N. (1989) 'Ethnography: Addressing the Practitioner', in J.F. Gubrium and D. Silverman (eds) *The Politics of Field Research*. London: Sage, pp. 197–212.

Capra, F. (1996) *The Web of Life*. London: Flamingo.

Carr, W. and Kemmis, S. (1986) *Becoming Critical: Education, Knowledge and Action Research*. London: Falmer Press.

Chendo, M. (2002) 'A Process Evaluation of Merseyside Health Action Zones: Funded Interventions and the Application of Capacity-Building Strategies at the District Level', M.Phil. thesis, unpublished.

Cohen, L. and Manion, L. (1984) 'Action Research', in J. Bell *et al.* (eds) *Conducting Small Scale Investigations in Educational Management*. London: Paul Chapman.

Cooke, B. and Kothari, U. (2001) *Participation: A New Tyranny*. London: Zed Books.

Dean, A. (1997) *Chaos and Intoxication*. London: Routledge.

Denzin, N.K. (1997) *Interpretive Ethnography: Ethnographic Practice for the 21st Century*. London: Sage.

Dunmore, N.L. (2002) 'Is Partnership Working? Perceptions and Experiences at the District Level of Merseyside Health Action Zone', M.Sc. thesis, unpublished.

Elden, M. and Levin, M. (1991) 'Co-generative Learning: Bringing Participation into Action Research', in W.F. Whyte (ed.) *Participatory Action Research*. London: Sage, pp. 127–41.

Fay, B. (1996) *Contemporary Philosophy of Social Science: A Multicultural Approach*. London: Blackwell.

Fisher, B., Neve, H. and Heritage, Z. (1999) 'Community Development, User Involvement, and Primary Health Care', *British Medical Journal* 318: 749–50.

Freire, P. (1970) *Pedagogy of the Oppressed*. New York: Herder and Herder.

Gardner, K. and Lewis, D. (1996) *Anthropology, Development and the Postmodern Challenge*. London: Pluto Press.

Greenwood, D.J. and Levin, M. (1998) *Introduction to Action Research: Social Research for Social Change*. London: Sage.

Gregory, R.L. (ed.) (1987) *The Oxford Companion to the Mind*. Oxford: Oxford University Press.

Hart, E. and Bond, M. (1995) *Action Research for Health and Social Care*. Buckingham: Open University Press.

Holter, I.M. and Schwartz-Barcott, D. (1993) 'Action Research: What Is It? How Has it Been Used and How Can it be Used in Nursing?', *Journal of Advanced Nursing* 18: 298–304.

Jayaratne, T.E. (1993) 'The Value of Quantitative Research for Feminist Research', in M. Hammersley (ed.) *Social Research: Philosophy, Politics and Practice*. London: Sage, pp. 109–123.

Kalleberg, R. (1990) *The Construct Turn in Sociology*. Oslo: Oslo Institute for Social Research.

De Koning, K. and Martin, M. (1996) *Participatory Research in Health*. London: Zed Books.

Lewin, K. (1948) 'Action Research and Minority Problems', in *Resolving Social Conflicts: Selected Papers in Group Dynamics*. New York: Harper Brothers.

Lincoln, Y.S. (1990) 'Fourth Generation Evaluation, the Paradigm Revolution, and Health Promotion', Keynote address, presented to the Health Promotion Research Methods: Expanding the Repertoire Conference, Toronto, Canada, 30–31 Dec.

Lincoln, Y.S. and Guba, E.G. (1985) *Naturalistic Inquiry*. London: Sage.

Macaulay, A.C., Commanda, L.E., Freeman, W.L., Gibson, N., McCabe, M.L., Robbins, C.M., Twohig, P.L. (1999) 'Participatory Research Maximises Community and Lay Involvement', *British Medical Journal* 319: 774–8.

Mies, M. (1993) 'Towards a Methodology for Feminist Research', in M. Hammersley (ed.) *Social Research: Philosophy, Politics and Practice*. London: Sage, pp. 64–82.

Mosse, D. (2001) ' "People's Knowledge", Participation and Patronage: Operations and Representations in Rural Development', in B. Cooke, R. Munck and D. O'Hearn (1999) *Critical Development: Contributions to a New Paradigm*. London: Zed Books.

Norgaard, R.B. (1994) *Development Betrayed: The End of Progress and a Coevolutionary Revisioning of the Future*. London: Routledge.

Oldham, J. and Rutter, I. (1999) 'Independence Days', *British Medical Journal* 318: 748–9.

Rahman, M.A. (1993) *People's Self Development: Perspectives on Participatory Action Research*. Guildford: Zed Books.

Reason, P. (1988) *Human Inquiry in Action: Developments in New Paradigm Research*. London: Sage.

Schutz, A. (1954) 'Concept and Theory Formation in the Social Sciences', *Journal of Philosophy* 51: 257–73.

Schwandt, T.A. (1994) 'Constructivist Interpretivist Approaches to Human Inquiry', in N.K. Denzin and Y.S. Lincoln (eds) *Handbook of Qualitative Research*. London: Sage.

Sokal, A. and Bricmont, J. (1998) *Intellectual Impostors*. London: Profile Books.

Springett, J. and Leavey, C. (1995) 'Participatory Action Research: The Development of a Paradigm, Dilemmas and Prospects', in N. Bruce, J. Springett, J. Hotchkiss and A. Scott-Samuel (eds) *Research and Change in Urban Community Health*. Aldershot: Avebury, pp. 57–66.

Stainton Rogers, W. (1991) *Explaining Health and Illness: An Exploration of Diversity*. London: Harvester Wheatsheaf.

Stringer, T. (1996) *Action Research: A Handbook for Practitioners*. London: Sage.

Tandon, R. (1993) 'The Historical Roots and Contemporary Tendencies in Participatory Research: Implications for Health Care', in K. de Koning and M. Martin (eds) *Participatory Research in Health*. London: Zed Books. pp. 19–23.

Thomas, P. (2002) 'Whole Systems Learning and Change in Primary Health Care – The Role of Primary Care Research Networks', M.D. thesis, unpublished.

Whyte, W.F. (ed.) (1991) *Participatory Action Research*. London: Sage.

Winter, R. (1989) *Learning from Experience: Principles and Practices in Action Research*. London: Falmer Press.

Zohar, D. (1991) *The Quantum Self*. London: Flamingo.

Zohar, D. and Marshall, I. (1993) *The Quantum Society: Mind, Physics and a New Social Vision*. London: Flamingo.

Chapter 4

Participation and empowerment in community care

Rowena Vickridge and Rosie Ayub

This chapter examines the way that health and social care organisations support patient and service user involvement in community care services. It develops this theme by describing some recent experience of supporting participation and involvement processes in Rochdale.

Community care involvement and consultation structures were formally established in response to the 1990 NHS and Community Care Act. Our experience in Rochdale has suggested that formal structures, while outwardly demonstrating the object and practice of patient and service user involvement, may actually limit or become a block to that process.

We argue that a model based on the principle of participation and empowerment is needed as a framework for understanding in what forms and at what levels involvement takes place. Applying this model in Rochdale has resulted in a move away from an emphasis on formal involvement structures and outcomes, towards recognising the importance of involvement processes. In practice this has meant a shift from static and formal, to fluid and informal, mechanisms.

The model which we describe below also provides a unifying framework for involvement at all levels of the organisation's activities, from service user contact with front-line staff to collective participation and influence in strategic and service planning.

Health promotion and community care

Where does involvement in community care services fit in with theories and practice of health promotion?

Social services have a longer tradition and more experience than their health partners in setting up involvement structures and processes. This is partly due to their location within local authority structures, which are framed within local democratic processes, and partly the remains of a thread deriving from the radical history of social work practice, which used community development and public participation methodologies during the 1970s and 1980s (Braye 2000; Thompson 2001). This contrasts with the traditional paternalism, more overt professional power structures and lack of public accountability that have often characterised healthcare organisations (Hugman 1991; Jones 1994).

Community care 'service users' represent some of the more vulnerable of the wider population of healthcare users. While healthcare services are likely to be used by the whole population at some life stage, only a minority of people will use social care services. Not all frail older people will come into contact with social care services, nor likewise disabled people, people with mental health issues, etc.

There is therefore a distinction between the wider population of, for example, older people, and the individual older service user who has direct experience of being assessed for, and receiving community care services. Health promotion activities, by contrast, may be directed at individuals and communities who belong within the larger group, and who may be living healthy active lives.

This chapter looks at the issues around involvement and participation in service planning and provision for users of community care services. However, the principles of autonomy, control and empowerment, which underpin the model described in this chapter, have equal relevance within the wider practice of health promotion, and rest on a community development methodology which has equal significance and currency.

Issues around service user involvement and empowerment are critical to other community care arenas – at the individual/professional interface within the assessment and care planning process; in the demand for development of user controlled and provided services in the form of direct payments. These other areas however warrant chapters in their own right, and within this text we focus primarily on service user involvement in strategic, as opposed to individual, service planning.

Health and social care policy: involvement and consultation

Since the 1990 NHS and Community Care Act, participation and involvement has been an underpinning theme in health and social care legislation and guidance.

Under the former Conservative government this was used to demonstrate a changed relationship between individual and the state, as expression of a 'contract culture' built on principles of the market and consumer choice. The Labour government in 1997 moved the emphasis from contract to partnership, and has subsequently issued a range of incentives and directives to make partnership the driver for modernisation at the local service and community level.

Both have sought to find evidence for this changed relationship within two distinct dynamics or processes. The first is at the individual patient or service user level, at the point of assessment of need and provision of service. The second is evidenced in the opportunities for individual or collective involvement in influencing the service planning process.

Both arenas for participation and involvement are contained within recent legislation and policy guidance. For example, the Health and Social Care Act 2001 puts in place the building blocks for what is termed 'our patient empowerment agenda'. New Patient Advocacy and Liaison Services, (PALS) and Patient Forums are the framework intended to drive the transformation of the relationship between NHS, patient and citizen, from an external accountability via Community Health Councils, to an integral involvement.

> Current structures relate to an outdated model whereby patients, carers and their representatives campaign to be heard from outside the NHS. It is our aim to ensure that ... the voices of citizens, patients and their carers are on the inside, influencing every level of service.
>
> (Department of Health [DoH] 2001:5)

Similarly the National Service Frameworks (NSFs) for coronary heart disease, cancer, mental health and older people demonstrate this new platform for the voice of patient/citizen within service planning and commissioning. These service frameworks all require evidence of patient and service user involvement in Local Implementation Teams, which are the vehicles responsible for meeting nationally applied standards and milestones.

In addition NSFs detail a more active role for patients and service users. For example, the NSF for older people sets out clear prescriptions, not only on 'person-centred care' (in relation to assessment and care planning), but also requires older people to be involved in the relevant 'Overview and Scrutiny Committee' to 'root out ageism' in locally applied policies and service criteria.

For local authorities, the Best Value Framework (Department of Environment 1998) requires a comprehensive and planned programme of service review, involving the development of procedures to consult with users of all local authority services, and the drawing up of local performance indicators to measure user satisfaction. Furthermore, the social services White Paper *Modernising Social Services* (1998) places partnership with users and carers at the centre of its programme for change. This requires full involvement of service users and carers in the development of social care charters, and that social services departments 'actively seek the views of the wider local community, including potential users and other stakeholders'.

Participation and the concept of empowerment

Although participation and empowerment are key themes in current health and social care policy, incorporating concepts of social inclusion, voice and control, they do not necessarily go hand in hand. Participation and involvement are often confused with empowerment. It is possible, however, and often the case, that involvement structures can be disempowering. At the same time, we argue, people using community care services do not have to be part of formal involvement structures for them to feel empowered and to have influence.

'The language of participation is complex: the same term means different things to different people, and the same concept may be known by a number of different terms' (Braye 2000: 9). For example, within a *consumerist model* (Croft and Beresford 1995) the term 'participation' can be used to describe one-off feedback via questionnaire as part of an organisation's measurement of customer satisfaction. Similarly, it can describe the use of surveys, focus groups and workshops, as a means of checking out predetermined policy and strategy in order to make it more relevant and flexible to the customer (or to give it a façade of user accountability [Carey 2000]).

By contrast the *democratic model* of participation sees the need and underlying purpose of involving service users in service planning as demonstrating the right of people to have a say in matters which affect them, and thereby to have greater control over their lives (Croft and Beresford 1995). As such it is related to concepts of citizenship and social inclusion. Within this model, the concept of empowerment sits more comfortably: '*Empowerment* ... means making it possible for people to exercise power and have more control over their lives. That means having a greater voice in institutions, agencies and situations, which affect them' (Croft and Beresford 1995: 62).

Yet the methodology of empowerment is itself heavily contested (Braye 2000). The dynamic between 'professional' and service user is critical: to some writers, empowerment is power that is taken rather than given. 'Power cannot be given but only taken, for to give power implies a gift from a position of power' (Jack 1995: 16). From this perspective, user groups need to challenge and claim power, and the professional, whose interests are to maintain his/her own power base, has a minor or non-existent role in supporting this process. Indeed, there is suspicion that professionals have colonised the empowerment agenda because of loss of autonomy within their own practice and a self-interested attempt to revitalise it through this platform (Baistow 1994; Croft and Beresford 1995; Jack 1995).

By contrast much of social work training has been underpinned by the belief that facilitation and empowerment are core social work skills. Thus Thompson's description of '*emancipatory practice*' (Thompson 2001) is located at two levels: first at an individual level in what he terms life politics; and, second, at a broader social inclusion level in emancipatory politics. The two, it is argued, are not mutually exclusive in that people may need to develop confidence and skills at a personal level before they can engage in a wider collective struggle. The social worker, within an underlying value framework of anti-discriminatory practice, needs to recognise and support this process. The challenge and required direction for the profession is to shift from a traditional paternalism to a relationship based on partnership with users, in what Hugman describes as 'democratic professionalism' (Hugman 1991).

Critics of those writers who makes claims for the value and significance of empowerment at the individual service user level argue that this dynamic is trapped within the structural inequality and imbalance of power between user and professional/welfare organisation. For example, Croft and Beresford describe the professional's interest in individual/personal empowerment as concerned with 'people taking increased responsibility for managing their lives, relationships and circumstances', which they equate with 'living in conformity with prevailing values and expectations, and to change in accordance with professionally set goals and norms' (1995: 63).

They contrast this with a 'liberational' model of empowerment, which is 'developed by movements of disabled people, older people and survivors and concerned with changing their position in society' (ibid.). Within this they allow for issues of personal empowerment but only 'in terms of ensuring people have the support, skills and personal resources they need for self organisation and participation to achieve broader social change' (ibid.).

The debate about the authenticity and significance of the personal and experiential has current parallels in disability studies and disability politics. Thomas reviews the debate between feminist writers and 'leading male social modellists'. The latter share a belief that:

> a focus on such matters (*the personal and experiential*) is diversionary: it saps the political energies of the disabled people's movement and bolsters oppressive models of disability (medical, individual, administrative).... Feminists, in contrast, reject forms of thought that posit a 'binary divide', that reproduce dualism, between the personal and the social. They see the social and political as just as present in the interstices and intimacies of day-to-day personal life, in the business of the 'private' dimensions of life, as it is in the 'public' domains of employment, education and other aspects of the wider social structure.
>
> (Thomas 2001: 49)

From our experience of involvement work in Rochdale we suggest that the individual and strategic/political levels are not mutually exclusive. We argue strongly for an understanding of 'agency' as an underpinning concept and believe that empowerment can be situational, – that an experience or situation where someone feels empowered can change the subsequent way that they interact with health and social care services. This correspondingly can impact on the service itself – through an interactive process driven at the small-scale and interpersonal level. This can be achieved without the service user necessarily getting involved at a 'higher' level to change services. We argue, however, that systems must be in place to recognise and support this process, since without the means of accumulating and registering these smaller-scale struggles or individual achievements, they would otherwise have no impact beyond the immediate.

If we talk about empowerment in the context of involvement, the model developed from work and experience in Rochdale views empowerment as a journey. Not a journey which necessarily starts at one set point and finishes at another, but a process of many different situations where people have the opportunity to build on skills, knowledge and experiences and put them to use at different times. People may also find the most empowering situation for them to voice their views is at a given place on that journey. However, most involvement structures are geared only to representation and participation at the formal and strategic level.

We also believe that concepts of empowerment should not be restricted to service users but that if the right process is facilitated well, workers should equally be empowered. Rather than viewing empowerment as a 'zero-sum' game (Barnes and Walker 1996), where empowerment claimed by one party is lost to the other, we believe that empowerment can derive from an active and mutual exchange dynamic. From this perspective, 'empowerment can give progressive substance to the exchange implicit in partnership' (Ward 2000: 51), where power is 'not obscured but viewed as a positive concept and used proactively by each party to promote his/her own interests and respond to the other's in the encounter' (Braye and Preston-Shoot 1995: 118). The basis of empowerment in the involvement process rests on recognising and valuing each other's distinctive knowledge or experience. We have found that it is often only when professionals have experienced really positive empowering involvement that they will move on to seek out and support more opportunities.

Ward suggests the potential of user groups, and groupwork as the vehicle for self-actualisation *and* empowerment, within the context of collectively expressed interests and issues. According to Ward, groups have a 'transformative capacity', as well as achieving material changes and raising the confidence of their members. Within this perspective the professional works in partnership with people, as facilitator rather than leading the process of decision making. Partnership and collaboration within the transformative capacity of the group process enables people to mobilise their creative potential.

The social action model described by Ward and focused on groupwork settings and processes, is closely allied to the community development approach inspired by the work of Paulo Freire (1972). Empowerment is a central theme in community development, and the relationship between community and worker is usually seen as less problematic than that between service user and professional. The community development approach starts with where the community is, unlike user involvement, in which involvement structures are often established not by practitioners but by policy makers. Imposing involvement structures with the appearance of user representation without the grassroots work to support this can lead to tokenistic practice, which produces a façade of participation and accountability. A top-down approach to participation and involvement can isolate and disempower service users, and the resulting drop-out rate is often blamed on the intrinsic difficulty of engaging with users rather than leading to an examination of the processes that are needed to provide a framework for partnership and collaboration.

Our aim here is to suggest how we can integrate participation and empowerment as a way of planning health and social care services. We believe that involvement is not beneficial to either providers or service users if it does not support the empowerment process.

We describe below a model setting out some of the practical aspects and issues needing to be addressed when organisations seek to support the empowerment process when involving service users. We do this to encourage and support practitioners, in the hope of enabling them 'to move from the inaction of endless conceptualisation into facilitating real change amongst groups of service users – without requiring superhuman skills or inexhaustible resources' (Ward and Mullender 1991: 24).

The model in Figure 4.1 depicts a journey which ranges from participation and involvement at an individual level, right through to service planning at the strategic level via individual or collective involvement in the planning process.

These two particular interfaces between the service user and community care organisations are significant in assessing the reality of the partnership relationship (power balance, equality and dynamic) between health and social care services and the individual. Between the two lies a whole range of different stages or levels at which participation and empowerment can take place. These different levels of involvement will be explored below with illustrations drawn from recent practice examples in Rochdale.

A model of participation and empowerment

Figure 4.1 introduces a model that we have used in Rochdale to understand the full range of opportunities which exist to hear the views of service users and explore the most appropriate means for people to get involved in the planning and delivery of community care services. This model aims to open up the involvement process to ensure that views at many different levels are heard. The importance of the model is that it prioritises the starting point for involvement at the place where people are already engaging with services or indeed with other service users. The model does not emphasise formal involvement structures as the way forward but stresses the need to value service users' informal structures and allow involvement processes to evolve where and how service users feel is most useful. For us the model symbolises the journey of involvement, where there is no set starting or finishing point. Many people will engage and get involved with services at only one point, while others will move through different levels gaining skills, knowledge and experience as they do so. Below is an explanation of what each level signifies and why it can be important.

Level 1 – individual service users and carers

This point in the journey is often the first contact that users have with community care services. Most people at this stage have no consistent method of ensuring their voice is heard in relation to changing and developing services. The way individuals experience contact at this level is vital, both for the individual and the service. The messages that the service gives at this point can either support the empowerment process or disempower the individual. For example, what choices are available? What information is passed on? What message is given about the openness of the organisation to feedback? Is advocacy offered? Our experience is that communication back to the organisation regarding users' views and ideas about services is often inconsistent and poorly developed at this level.

Level 2 – clubs, activity groups, drop-ins, social centres

Informal groups and networks are often important to service users. In these situations people feel able to talk and to share experiences, some of which are about services. It is at this point that we can learn from people who would never contemplate getting involved in formal structures. However, once people are aware that they can have an impact on services and have built relationships and trust with supporters of involvement, they are more likely to get involved in other groups and structures.

Level 3 – user groups, carers' groups, advocacy groups

Groups at this level are often user-led, or may be facilitated by someone independent of the service. The membership is mainly of service users. These groups may arise around shared interests or may be issue-related. They may be support or campaigning groups, and are often an indication that people have strong views about services and related issues. Engaging with groups at this level is vital to the involvement process. It can give a clear indication of the issues which are important to service users and how people wish to be involved.

Level 4 – operational groups

This level identifies those groups which take place around a specific service such as a day centre, for example. Stakeholders in the day centre would have representation in this group, including staff and service users. This is a more immediate kind of involvement and represents an important point in the journey of involvement and empowerment. The skills, knowledge and experience that can be gained at this stage are vital and it is often from these processes that people go on to get more involved at a strategic level.

Level 5 – joint working (partnership) groups

This level indicates joint working at a wider service level, for example, drawing representatives from the whole of the mental health service. It is at this level that views and ideas about future developments within the service are discussed, and it is often the place where user representation becomes recognised and formalised. It is therefore vital that service users feel empowered to engage in these groups. It is also important, however, that users' views expressed through other channels are fed back at this level to impact on developments.

Level 6 – strategic planning groups and level 7 – decision making group

These represent strategic planning and decision making groups (for example the NSF Local Implementation Teams), and it is important that service users are represented at these levels. There is however often little thought about what is needed to support this involvement to make it effective rather than tokenistic. There are issues which need to be considered relating to the potential for isolation and a need for strong links to a wider constituency of service users.

Level 8 – other consultation and involvement forums

This represents the links which need to exist with the wider network of involvement structures within local authority, health bodies, local strategic partnership, etc. This level of involvement moves from single issue or service level to wider corporate planning, and represents an important platform for involvement around socially inclusive strategies on, for example, disability equality issues.

Characteristics of the model

- Each level represents opportunities for varied and fluid participation and empowerment. There is no relative value ascribed to different levels, and people can engage at any point.

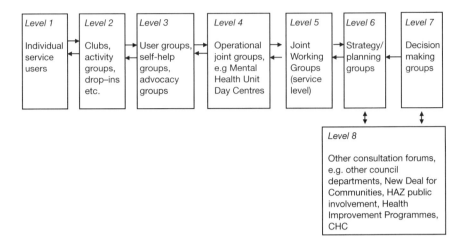

Figure 4.1 A model of participation and involvement

- More service users are present from level 1 and numbers decrease as we move towards level 7. This needs to be illustrated in the way we involve people to ensure users are valued at every level.
- The consultation context becomes more formalised as it progresses from level 1 to level 7. Attention needs to be paid to ensure that the views and ideas in the early stages of the model are not lost.
- Many people may not wish or are not able to engage in the groups illustrated in levels 4–7.
- It is usually the case that fewer resources are targeted at the involvement of people from levels 1–4. This balance needs to change if we are to ensure an open fluid process.
- Service users who do engage in levels 4–7 can either become isolated or entrenched if there are no links with levels 1–3.

If we are to shift the culture of consultation and involvement, we need to ensure that the organisation as a whole is supporting the empowerment process. This means examining the organisational culture to identify how far it encourages or limits participation across the whole spectrum of levels described above. It also means developing creative approaches to involvement to ensure we reach the 'silent majority' of service users, and avoid putting too great an emphasis on more traditional methods that prioritise structures and outcomes as opposed to processes. Using a community development approach helps build the capacity of service users and user groups to engage on their own terms, and ensures that groups and processes are sustainable in the long term. Staff need training and support so that they become more proactive in the involvement process. And, finally, attention needs to be paid to establishing an effective communication process, to adopt an 'open ear' policy that listens in a continuous way to people where they are already talking and sharing their views about services.

We examine below in more detail the points raised above.

Key themes and issues

The culture of the organisation

There are tensions and conflicting interests within public service organisations between managerial and professional values and practices. (Newman and Clarke 1994). Empowering practice with service users requires a degree of worker/professional autonomy, which sits uncomfortably with strict managerial control over standardised procedures, targets and quantifiable performance measurement. This latter is itself a necessary response to an increasingly centralised control over performance and standards in health and social care services by government, measuring efficiency through externally imposed targets and providing financial rewards or penalties linked to ratings on published league tables. The prevailing culture of 'naming and shaming' has consequences for the ethos of public service organisations and the morale of workers within them. It has been argued that the 'accountability revolution', as well as distorting professional/organisational practice, also corrodes the potential for openness and trust (O'Neill, 2002).

However, the practice of collaborative and partnership working, between agencies, different groups of professionals, and professionals/ service users, in itself both requires and generates an openness to new ways of working, based on mutual learning rather than on prescription of outcome. The skills needed for partnership working emphasise the equal worth of participants and the value derived from the diversity of experience, both between users and professionals and across the health and social service traditions.

The model of participation and involvement we describe requires an organisational culture that recognises and values front-line staff. It emphasises the importance of the dynamic or process at initial contact or through individual working relationships. It requires that staff themselves are empowered, involved in decision making, have a voice which is heard, are given a supported autonomy, encouraged to use initiative and receive positive reinforcement. In our experience, once staff do engage with involvement processes, the experience of 'doing things differently' can bring about changes in practice.

Involving front-line staff

Although assessment teams and front-line staff should be at the very heart of involvement, their contribution and potential is often unrecognised. We need to build on the relationships of trust which often exist at this level, to listen to what people are saying about service issues and feed this back into the organisation.

Many of the staff in our organisations are creative, enthusiastic and have skills and experience outside of their present roles. Many of these staff can clearly see where more innovative approaches and projects would have a long-term benefit for their service users, but are not encouraged to develop these if they step outside of current practice and routine demands of the service. New projects often go to outside sources or new staff. This undermines and devalues staff. Organisations and services users are losing out by not being more creative in the way they use their present workforce, especially those who are motivated to try out their ideas. This is also the case for many service users who have rich life experiences other than those of using services.

Two recent examples of the front-line initiatives in Rochdale are given below.

A social worker and two service users of a neuro-rehabilitation unit at the local hospital have recently set up a support group for young people with physical or cognitive impairments ('Kick-start'). They were aware that when people left the unit they were isolated and often housebound. The group immediately attracted forty members and is still growing. The outcomes from the group have been impressive, not only in terms of mutual support and increasing confidence, but through the networks they have established. The group is beginning to engage with different services, seek out the support which members need and find shared solutions to problems. While essentially a support group with no expressed interest in formal involvement channels, the group will be included in any future consultation process, on its own terms and 'turf'. Groupwork facilitation skills have been essential to developing the confidence and sustainability of the group, but also the inter-personal knowledge and trust of both social worker and members were needed as a starting point.

In a second example of using the potential strengths of front-line staff in involvement, the 'Have your Say' project has worked with a group of home care staff to reach and listen to the views of older housebound people, who make up part of the 'silent majority' of service users. This pilot project is part of the local implementation of the National Service Framework for Older People, which is supporting new ways of involving older people. We felt it important to ensure that we were involving those older people who were not able to attend meetings and forums. We wanted to explore ways to hear the views of the most vulnerable people. Many of these people use the homecare service and have built up good relationships with workers. Homecare workers routinely hear people's views and experiences of many different services, for example, district nursing, day care, hospital services as well as those relating to homecare itself. Although care workers are often the people to whom these views are informally expressed, there is no consistent way of feeding them in to the planning process. As to the care workers, they are unsure how to respond, or what to do with information which falls outside the official complaints procedure.

We wanted to explore how we could support the homecare workers to take on more of a listening role with clients. The other strand to the project was to offer more creative options for giving feedback e.g. face-to-face with workers or managers, through the use of a video camera, by computer or dictaphone, or through an advocate. Training sessions were provided for homecare workers in areas such as listening skills and basic interviewing techniques. The homecare workers were also involved in the process of developing information leaflets about the project and in designing the semi-structured questionnaire. Their experience and knowledge was invaluable in these processes. While the project is still under way at present, what has emerged so far is their enthusiasm and growing confidence in playing a key role in enabling the voices of service users and carers to be heard by senior managers. In a similar way to the first example, the personal knowledge and trust between care worker and older person has been a vital link in the project.

Structure versus process

As stated earlier, current guidance on health and social care services requires demonstrable representation and involvement in formal joint planning structures. In addition, the Health and Social Care Act 2001 sets out the future configuration of patient involvement structures from local to regional and national level. Guidance also specifies what form this should take, for example, the new Patients' Forums.

In principle this ensures that consultation and partnership takes on a new emphasis and weight within health and social care, and this is to be welcomed. However, our experience suggests that if we are to ensure that involvement supports empowerment, establishing 'top-down' structures could actually hinder this objective, unless attention is given to the wider process of partnership working.

This has been a finding of our recent review of Rochdale's Partnership Groups. These were set up as part of the community care joint planning structures following the NHS and Community Care Act 1990, as the formal consultation and involvement forums for all community care service areas (mental health, older people, learning disabilities, disabled people, drugs and alcohol, and children). These groups were innovative and forward-thinking at the time they were established, and demonstrated a visible commitment to user involvement. They also now provide evidence of some of the limitations inherent in formalised structures, which can prevent real empowerment from taking place.

First, the groups were large and made up of a mainly professional membership. They only had a few long-standing service user and carer members, mostly no longer directly using services. The groups were the formal channel for consultation when user involvement was needed for strategic or service development decisions, however they had very few links with the wider service user and carer population. There were no resources directed at involvement at a grassroots level. The main body of service users were either unaware of the existence of the groups, or did not wish to get involved because they saw them as professionally dominated. Many formal structures like the Partnership Groups continue to use long-standing user and carer representatives who have long been involved and have learnt to conform/fit in with the way professionals meet and make decisions. Representation can become tokenistic, and individuals can be expected to comment on services they know little about.

Second, the process of establishing 'top-down' formal structures already excludes how service users would choose to get involved, and hence there is no guarantee that involvement will be empowering. The review of the Partnership Groups by users concluded that meetings were too large, venues and times were not always conducive to involving new people, and they were too formal. Service users who were involved also felt that they did not have access to the same resources as the professionals, and that written information was presented in an inaccessible language or to unrealistic deadlines which limited their ability to fully participate.

Finally, by putting the emphasis on structures, the likelihood is that the process of participation will be overlooked. Since the Partnership Groups were established, no time had been given to how the groups would actually work in partnership. Ground rules were not explored and set, and issues about how different parties would respond to conflicting viewpoints were not identified. When a group is top-heavy with professionals, unless these issues are explored, it makes it harder for service users to challenge the way things are done.

The Partnership Groups have played an important role from the organisations' perspective, in terms of profile, structure, formality and convenience, all of which aspects help manage consultation requirements within an increasingly complex national and local policy agenda. However, the review carried out confirms that they have failed to meet the needs of users/carer members on an equal level, nor have they helped create a channel for the views of the wider membership of service users.

Community development approach

The key themes underlying a community development approach are empowerment, capacity-building and sustainability. We believe that, by taking a community development approach to involvement, we can address many of the issues that are raised by our model. Capacity-building means ensuring that we work at a grassroots level, to get people involved and support them with training, resources, etc. Building capacity also needs to have regard to supporting ways of sustaining that involvement. This may mean supporting service users to seek out their own funding rather than to rely on statutory services, ensuring the group's independence, control and continuity.

To support capacity-building in Rochdale we have ensured that involvement budgets have been redirected to support the work of developing the grassroots level groups. While some of this work has been facilitated by front-line staff (as described above), most has been provided through contracts with external agencies and workers to give support to emerging groups. The success of this has been two-fold. First, it has given groups the financial and organisational support they desperately needed to develop and, second, it has provided a degree of independence from statutory services.

When groups of service users do evolve, they can begin to shift the culture of involvement further by demanding a seat at the table, pushing for professionals to meet them on their terms, supporting other service users to get involved, and having a group mandate when representing views.

Between July 2001 to March 2002, grassroots development work linked to participation and involvement has taken place in five different areas: with drug and alcohol users, mental health service users, parents of disabled children, older people, and learning disabled people. Some of these groups are now moving towards seeking independent funding, and user control and management. A mental health service user group in Rochdale has been given funding to set up a user-managed resource, including an office, computer, use of telephone, etc. The parents group has seen direct outcomes of their involvement in improving access to mainstream leisure facilities, and is in the process of broadening its membership and influence.

As an example of the process of establishing groups, we describe recent work with people who use drug and alcohol services. Previous to this there was no user involvement in this service area, despite the formally established, and professionally attended, drug and alcohol Partnership Group equivalent.

As described in the model in Figure 4.1, many people who use services are already meeting in a variety of ways and settings. They are often already engaged in informal interest and client groups, such as meeting in a 'drop in'. These informal groups are the ideal place to explore with service users how they might wish to get involved in changing services. Resources need to be directed at this level to support capacity-building and to give people the opportunity and time to test out ideas.

On visiting and listening to drug and alcohol users in various settings around Rochdale, a number of issues emerged. First, people were very cynical about whether anything they did say would be taken seriously because of the stigma attached to drugs and alcohol users. Contrary to the view of professionals that anything service users wanted would cost money, it emerged that attitudes of professionals and the way services were provided was of far more importance to users.

Although many users did want to have a say about services, it took a long time for a collective approach to be agreed. What emerged was a small group who wanted to broaden user representation within drug and alcohol services. The setting up of this group was a long process. Different times and venues were tried out and the aims of the group regularly revisited, taking some considerable time before these felt right for everyone. Some people could only attend the group a few times, and it was important to have no preconceptions about regular or consistent attendance, because some of the short-term members played an important part in helping move the group on. The best way to build the capacity of a group is for the users to run and control it and to recruit its members. However, experience here proved that people were glad of allies, that is, workers who are familiar with services and can support them in negotiating with providers.

One of the lessons learnt from this experience was to avoid preconceived ideas about how a group will develop, and assumptions about the numbers of people who want to get involved. For many people this will be the first time they have even considered using their experiences to change services. Going back to groups time and again, even if just to share a cup of tea and exchange ideas, was an important part of the process.

Alongside setting up the group, it was necessary to work with professionals in drug and alcohol services and seek out further allies. Supporting staff to understand how and why people who use services need to be involved and consulted is vital.

The service users made clear how they wished to be involved in the future. They asked for members of their group to sit on the interagency Drug and Alcohol Reference Group, and on the Alcohol Strategy Group. The service users also felt that it was important to have dialogue with service providers in a way that suited them. They negotiated with a number of managers for them to attend their user group bi-monthly. This group continues to meet and has asked for support in compiling an information leaflet. It has also recently sent a representative to a national conference, and members have now made links with other projects and networks.

Service user and worker champions

Champions inside and outside the organisation, who understand and seek partnership and collaboration opportunities, are essential to helping promote and support involvement and empowerment, and to ensure that it becomes a real process. Staff and managers inside the organisation can help continue to promote involvement. Individual service users are more likely to get the support from other service users to extend influence. People have more confidence in trusting someone who they feel understands their position, and has likewise had experience of using services. In Rochdale, partnership and empowerment champions have emerged both inside and outside the health and social care organisations. The impact of this has been important in moving from a position where involvement is seen as the responsibility of one lead involvement worker to a much broader approach involving a network of people, groups/structures and projects, shaping the way involvement processes develop.

Importance of training

When training is discussed around involvement, it is usually seen as patients or service users needing to be given training in how to participate in meetings. This can suggest an unintentionally patronising and one-sided learning process, which emphasises and reinforces inequalities in relative status and power. By contrast, we have found that it is often staff who need to acquire different skills to work in a collaborative way with users in meetings.

Training is also an important means of breaking through the traditional paternalism of professionals and care workers, to develop a culture which is based on partnership and collaboration, and which recognises and values the expertise of direct experience. This gives the message that we all have knowledge and expertise in our fields and that this includes the direct experience of using services.

In Rochdale, a group including mental health service users was successful in submitting an application to a regional training fund to provide training to both staff and service users. It was very important that both groups were involved as participants in joint sessions and also in some sessions where service users provided the training. This joint training also provided opportunities to hear each other's perspective regarding involvement and to ensure that each group was witness to the commitments proposed by the other.

Other aims of the training included finding more creative approaches to involvement, building the capacity of service users, which would increase the number of people who wished to get involved, as well as providing training to give people the necessary confidence, skills and knowledge that they felt they needed. Through a 'training the trainers' course we are aiming to establish a pool of local service user trainers who could be bought in to provide training to other service users and professionals.

In another project, an external co-ordinator is working with a group of older people to establish a training programme around identifying ageism and anti-discriminatory practice. This will be used within staff training sessions in a variety of health and social care settings, starting with sessions provided for care staff in a local nursing home.

In a similar way, a programme of disability equality training is to be rolled out to all assessment and care staff, purchased from and facilitated by an organisation of disabled people.

Including external groups and organisations

We have found that a collaborative approach to developing policy and strategy requires agencies to be open to as wide a range of user views and perspectives as possible. This may extend beyond the scope of 'internal' service user experience to include external user-led groups and organisations.

In developing Rochdale's Strategy for Physical and Sensory Impairment, the early involvement of the Disabled People's Working Party (DPWP) within the steering group introduced a clear value base, established on principles of independent living and the social model of disability, which underpinned the strategy from the outset. This resulted in a coherent strategy and action plan affecting all aspects of the way services were provided to disabled people. It helped move service provision from that based on the traditional segregated model, to supporting independent living in personal care (through direct payments), accommodation, and access to mainstream employment and education. The DPWP existed as a consultation group on corporate disability issues in the local authority, rather than as a group of users of health and social care services. It is unlikely that this explicit value base and policy direction would have been reached without the involvement of the DPWP. It demonstrated the importance of working within the wider framework of rights, citizenship and social inclusion, and not to limit partnership to the potentially narrower scope of service user concerns and experience.

Monitoring and scrutiny

If groups and individuals are involved in strategic and service development, systems need also to be in place to ensure that progress towards agreed strategies or action plans can be monitored. For example, a Reference Group has been established to monitor progress on the Strategy for Physical and Sensory Impairment, made up of a group of disabled people who came together from a one-off consultation exercise around the strategy. This group now meets every three months to monitor the progress of the strategy.

Officers are expected to provide written progress reports to the group, as well as attending when requested. The group has a very clear remit, and provides a challenging forum for agencies if progress is not in line with that promised in the strategy. At the same time, involving service users in scrutiny provides the opportunity for reviewing and reassessing priorities in a transparent way if resources do not allow services to reach action plan targets.

This means that people involved have a better understanding and insight into budget and resource constraints, and can work collectively to agree priorities or alter time scales.

Developing quality standards

The performance of health and social care agencies is increasingly the subject of measurement and audit. The stated purpose is to provide national standards to provide a framework for, and therefore shape, practice, as well as developing quantifiable and nationally comparable outcomes. One of the issues related to performance assessment and evaluation is that measurable and quantifiable outcomes may not capture the qualitative aspects of service provision, which often better express the concerns of people who use services (Nocon and Qureshi 1996).

It is important, therefore, that agencies involve users in developing standards which express quality of outcome, as well as, for example, service activity rates. This presents a challenge to organisations which are struggling to meet the demands of the 'audit explosion' (O'Neill 2002). However, we suggest that quality issues can and should be addressed within practice through bottom-up initiatives which learn from the collaboration and experience of practitioners *and* service users.

For example, nursing and social work practitioners in a Rochdale hospital worked together in a project to improve practice around the care and hospital discharge arrangements of palliative care patients (Vickridge 1998). Written guidelines were established which became part of hospital protocol and were monitored by clinical audit. Crucial to this work was the involvement of service users, who made significant contributions to the guidelines, particularly around how the medical diagnoses should be communicated to patient and family.

We have found that many of the issues for users are as much about *the way* in which services are provided as about resources. These are difficult to measure because they relate to qualities such as dignity, respect, communication, trust and continuity. A 'person-centred' service, which the government's health reforms promise, must also incorporate standards which reflect these aspects.

Communication process

For the model in Figure 4.1 to work, it is essential that there is a communication strategy in place to which the organisation and its partners sign up. This would seek to ensure that views of service users at every level were collected and channelled to feed in to service review and development. We need to adopt a culture of continual listening, that is, an 'open ear' policy. This means that we find ways to listen to what people are saying, when and where they are saying it, and more appropriate ways to gather and collate that information without necessarily creating new structures and forums.

Communication is an essential part of an empowering process. If people's views are expressed, but the outcomes of their involvement are not communicated back to them, this disempowers and devalues anyone who has given their time to get involved. Service users become cynical about consultation events which seek views, but which lead to no apparent change. Sometimes this is simply because no one has taken responsibility for communicating the outcomes.

Furthermore, all too often groups and meetings which involve people remain outside of the main key strategic and decision making groups, and there is a lack of clarity about reporting arrangements and spheres of influence. It is important that there are clear routes for channelling views in all involvement work, otherwise service users feel that their participation is devalued and their time wasted.

Partnership working

Bringing people together with different perspectives and agendas, and expecting people to reach joint solutions, is not easy. Involving service users in this process adds a new dimension. Very often little thought is given to the group process, to ensure that people not only listen to different perspectives, but are also able to appreciate and value them in a way that facilitates a move to joint solutions.

Often it is the most powerful or confident individuals in the group who will dominate the direction. Involving service users frequently means that, although they have a seat at the table, their voice is not heard. Any partnership group of this kind, in the initial phase of setting up, should prioritise taking time to consider the process and to set joint ground rules. This exercise would not only enable the group to work on an equal basis but would also nurture an environment of trust where difficult issues can be tackled.

Funding involvement

Organisations must make resources available to support user involvement and participation. We have found, however, that compared with other areas of service, relatively small budgets can make a huge difference in involvement work. Making available resources such as meeting space, office space and equipment, and administrative support, which organisations often take for granted, are relatively low cost but make a big contribution to 'start-up' costs for groups.

We have also found that user groups benefit from dedicated support in their initial stages, and that this can often be best provided by buying in the time of external and independent agencies or workers. Again, this has not proved to be a large cost commitment, but it has had an enormous impact in terms of developing capacity and broadening the basis for participation and involvement. In the longer term, groups can be assisted with applications for external funding to ensure they become financially independent of services.

Strategic direction and co-ordination

Finally, we suggest that organisations develop a clear interagency strategy for involvement and consultation, which is signed up to by health and social care partnership boards, as well as having named involvement leads at senior management level.

In Rochdale, an interagency strategy has been developed to give direction and clarity to involvement work. Its recommendations are now to be implemented through a user-directed Joint Steering Group. It aims to bring involvement work into a coherent whole, and sets criteria against which any consultation or involvement should be judged. Because of the plethora of consultation requirements within local authorities and healthcare organisations, it is important that there be a shared agreement about the purpose and standards for involvement as well as co-ordination of involvement processes and initiatives.

Conclusions

In conclusion, we take issue with the reductionist and adversarial models of involvement which see professionals and workers as being located in oppressive power relations with service users. We suggest that these models do not reflect the fluidity of interests and opportunities for individuals, both internal and external, to organisations. Neither do they take account of the way in which individuals can inhabit simultaneously or move easily between different roles and relationships. For example, paid workers/professionals may also simultaneously be service users and/or carers in their own right. Similarly, service users may also be employers of care staff (using direct payments). Notions of power and empowerment therefore need to be relative and fluid rather than absolute and fixed.

We suggest that this government's emphasis on collaboration and partnership should have equal resonance within organisations, in terms of needing to value front-line staff, and that an organisation which values and empowers staff will also be one which puts in place the opportunities to involve and empower service users.

The model of empowerment we describe gives equal value to different 'levels' of involvement, from service users mobilising around isolated or 'one-off' concerns and issues, to formal collaboration in strategic planning. While organisations may demonstrate support for the latter, they often ignore opportunities to build capacity at grassroots level or to use the potential of existing informal user groups and networks.

How do we know if an empowering culture is working? Not by quantifying the sum of participation, because participation can exist without empowerment. Equally, user support groups can exist which are excluded from the decision making process and therefore have no impact on services. The measure of success would be in the existence of independent and self-sustaining groups which are separate from, but participants in, decision making at all levels, and an open organisation within which empowerment is everyone's business.

References

Baistow, K. (1994) 'Liberation and Regulation: Some Paradoxes of Empowerment', *Critical Social Policy* 14(3): 34–46.

Barnes, M. and Walker, A. (1996) 'Principles of Empowerment', *Policy and Politics* 24(4): 375–93.

Braye, S. (2000) 'Participation and Involvement in Social Care', in H. Kemshall and R. Littlechild (eds) *User Involvement and Participation in Social Care*. London: Jessica Kingsley p.9.

Braye, S. and Preston-Shoot, M. (1995) *Empowering Practice in Social Care*. Buckingham: Open University Press.

Carey, P. (2000) 'Community Health Promotion and Empowerment', in J. Kerr (ed.) *Community Health Promotion, Challenges for Practice*. London: Balliere Tindall, Harcourt.

Croft, S. and Beresford, P. (1995) 'Whose Empowerment? Equalising the Competing Discourses in Community Care', in R. Jack (ed.) *Empowerment in Community Care*. London: Chapman Hall.

Department of the Environment, Transport and the Regions (1998) *Improving Local Services through Best Value*. London: HMSO.

Department of Health (2001) *Involving Patients and the Public in Healthcare: A Discussion Document*. London: DoH p.5

Department of Health (1998) *Modernising Social Services: Promoting Independence, Improving Protection, Raising Standards, Cm 4169*. London: The Stationery Office.

Freire, P. (1972) *Pedagogy of the Oppressed*. Harmondsworth: Penguin.

Hugman, R. (1991) *Power in Caring Professions*. London: Macmillan.

Jack, R. (1995) 'Empowerment in Community Care', in R. Jack (ed.) *Empowerment in Community Care*. London: Chapman Hall.

Jones, L. (1994) *The Social Context of Health and Health Work*. London: Macmillan.

Newman, J. and Clarke, J. (1994) 'Going about Our Business? The Managerialization of Public Services', in J. Clarke, A. Cochrane and E. McLaughlin (eds) *Managing Social Policy*. London: Sage.

Nocon, A. and Qureshi, H. (1996) *Outcomes of Community Care for Users and Carers*. Buckingham: Open University Press.

O'Neill, A. (2002) 'A Question of Trust', 2002 Reith Lectures, BBC.

Thomas, C. (2001) 'Feminism and Disability: The Theoretical and Political Significance of the Personal and Experiential', in L. Barton (ed.) *Disability, Politics and the Struggle for Change*. London: David Fulton.

Thompson, N. (2001) *Anti-discriminatory Practice*. London: Palgrave Macmillan.

Turner, M. and Balloch, S. (2001) 'Partnership between Service Users and Statutory Social Services', in S. Balloch and M. Taylor (eds) *Partnership Working*. Bristol: Policy Press.

Vickridge, R. (1998) 'Collaborative Working for Good Practice in Palliative Care', *Journal of Interprofessional Care* 12(1): 63–7.

Ward D. (2000) ' Totem not Token: Groupworks as a Vehicle for User Participation' in H. Kemshall and R. Littlechild (eds) User Involvement and Participation in Social Care, London: Jessica Kingsley p.51.

Ward, D. and Mullender, A. (1991) 'Empowerment and Oppression: An Indissoluble Pairing for Contemporary Social Work', *Critical Social Policy* 32: 21–30.

Chapter 5

Social inclusion and inequalities in health

Grahame D. Wright

The purpose of this chapter is to examine how social policy has influenced the work of health promotion, particularly in the last decade. During this time the government has developed health strategies which have been designed to improve the health of the population in Britain. Early health strategies did not acknowledge health inequalities and it was not until the New Labour government took office that this was addressed. In recent years it has been recognised that there are a number of sections of the community which are socially excluded for a variety of reasons. The government has produced policies in England, Scotland, Wales and Northern Ireland which are designed to deal with social exclusion and which have implications for local government. The focus of many of these strategies is the process of community development and the empowerment of local communities. The process of community development is complex, as is the process of empowerment, and it is not clear to what extent we can truly empower communities in the current political climate or whether we just enable people to improve their health.

When the New Labour government came to power they introduced a fresh policy for the delivery of healthcare in Britain (Department of Health [DoH] 1997) which was designed to eliminate competitive elements from the delivery of healthcare and instead, introduced co-operation between agencies. Health Improvement Plans are now an essential part of the provision for healthcare, which operates at local level. They are intended to encourage different agencies to work together to plan and deliver measures to improve the health of the population. Interagency working is essential if health improvement plans are to be successfully implemented. This means that stakeholders, such as local authorities, primary care and the voluntary sector should adopt a collaborative approach, which will address both healthcare issues and the wider determinants of health. For some this will be a new approach to promoting the health of the population and therefore it could be considered embryonic. If it works then this will shape the future of health promotion.

Health inequalities

Since the 1980s it has been recognised that inequalities in health exist in Britain and that this has had an effect on the mortality and morbidity rates. In 1977 the government established a working group on inequalities in health, chaired by Sir Douglas Black (Goldblatt and Whitehead 2000). Their report brought together evidence of inequalities in mortality, in long-standing illness and in the utilisation of health services (particularly preventive services). They concluded that there was no 'single and simple explanation' for these differences and that the predominant or governing explanation for inequalities in health lay in the material deprivation and specific features of the socio-economic environment. *The Black Report* (Black 1988), as it is now referred to, offered a structural explanation of health inequalities in as much as the social class gradient largely mirrored the extent to which people had access to the material determinants of health status, such as income, housing, education and safe working environments. Social policy therefore needed to be wide-ranging in order to address these issues. This is further supported by evidence provided by a follow-up study, which produced evidence that health inequalities were widening, especially among adults (Whitehead 1988). This was largely ignored by the government of the day and consequently health policies introduced in 1992 focused on the medical model of health and did not address the wider determinants of health.

Dahlgren and Whitehead (1991) identified that, while individuals are endowed with age, sex and constitutional factors, these are affected by individual lifestyle factors which, in turn, are influenced by social and community networks, which likewise are influenced by general socio-economic, cultural and environmental conditions. These include living and working conditions, such as the work environment, education, agriculture and food production, unemployment, water and sanitation, healthcare services and housing. Health inequalities are inextricably linked to life circumstances in many ways.

The aim of social policy is to improve human welfare and to meet human needs for education, health, housing and social security, areas identified in health inequalities. Bunton (in Bunton and McDonald 1992) reports that health promotion professes to be centrally concerned with the social policy process. Building healthy public policy is one of the five means of health promotion action to achieve Health For All by the year 2000 – along with, creating supportive environments, strengthening community action, developing personal skills and reorienting health services. These are the five areas for action listed in the *Ottawa Charter* (WHO 1986). Two good examples of healthy public policy in Britain over the last decade are embodied in *The Health of the Nation* (DoH 1992) and in *Scotland's Health: A Challenge to Us All* (Scottish Office Department of Health [SOHD] 1992). Although health inequalities had been identified in the 1980s, neither of these policy statements acknowledged the importance of addressing the determinants of health. This meant that health promotion focused on topics such as heart disease, stroke and cancer. There was a particular focus on lifestyles, implicitly assuming that a change in behaviour would guarantee perfect health. It is now generally accepted that this is not the case and that health is also determined to a great extent by our environment and social circumstances. It is widely recognised that poverty is associated with poor health, even in rich societies. In order to develop policies to tackle health inequalities we need to be much clearer about the relationship between specific dimensions of socio-economic circumstances and health (Benzeval *et al.* 2000). The Labour government acknowledges that life circumstances play an important part in the health of the population.

In 1998 Sir Donald Acheson instigated an independent inquiry into inequalities in health. The result of this inquiry recommended that government health policies should be evaluated in terms of their impact on health inequalities. This is strongly emphasised in current policies on health such as *Saving Lives: Our Healthier Nation* and *Towards a Healthier Scotland* (DoH 1999; SOHD 1999a). *Our Healthier Nation* (DoH 1998a) addressed issues of the physical and social environment – neighbourhoods, community safety, transport, access to high-quality health and social services, and poverty, employment and social exclusion were identified as specific socio-economic factors affecting health. Similar documents exist in Northern Ireland and in Wales. All of these policies are intended to guide the work of health promotion.

Sir Donald Acheson endorsed a socio-economic model to explain health inequalities. His report emphasises the interactions between lifestyle and wider influences on health such as economic, cultural and environmental conditions. He states that:

> Socio-economic inequalities in health reflect differential exposure – from before birth and across the lifespan – to risks associated with socio-economic position. These differential exposures are also important in explaining health inequalities, which exist by ethnicity and gender.
>
> (Acheson 1998: 6)

He further states that:

> we have therefore recommended both 'upstream' and 'downstream' policies – those which deal with wider influences on health inequalities, such as income distribution, education, public safety, housing, work, employment, social networks, transport and pollution, as well as those which have a narrower impacts, such as healthy behaviours.
>
> (Acheson 1998: 8)

Graham (1999) observed that getting the balance right is far from simple:

> Reductions in health inequalities represent 'downstream' solutions which require strategies which target 'upstream' influences. How to equalise access to the determinants of good health is likely to be a question framed by disagreements about evidence, both on causal pathways and on effective solutions.

In order to deal with health inequality there needs to be a commitment from national and local agencies. Through interagency working and a long-term strategy it is possible that tackling inequality will become a reality. One of the key aims of the government's health strategy for England is to improve the health of the worst-off in society and to narrow the health gap.

Social exclusion

The term 'social exclusion' originated in the social policy of the French socialist governments of the 1980s. It was used to refer to a disparate group of people living on the margins of society and, in particular, those without access to the system of social insurance.

Social exclusion has been defined by the European Commission as follows:

> Social exclusion refers to the multiple and changing factors resulting in people being excluded from the normal exchanges, practices and rights of modern society. Poverty is one of the most obvious factors, but social exclusion also refers to inadequate rights in housing, education, health and access to services. It affects individuals and groups, particularly in urban and rural areas, who are in some way subject to discrimination or segregation, and it emphasises the weaknesses in the social infrastructure and the risk of allowing a two-tier society to become established by default. The Commission believes that a fatalistic acceptance of social exclusion must be rejected, and that all community citizens have a right to the respect of human dignity.
>
> (Commission of the European Communities 1993, cited in
> Percy-Smith 2000: 3)

Percy-Smith explains that:

> In the U.K. the concept of social exclusion came with the setting up by the government in 1997 of the interdepartmental Social Exclusion Unit. The Social Exclusion Unit only encompasses England: social exclusion and poverty are devolved responsibilities and, in Scotland there is a

separate 'Scottish Social Inclusion Strategy'; in Wales 'Building an Inclusive Wales'; and in Northern Ireland 'Targeting Social Need in Northern Ireland'.

(Percy-Smith 2000)

The Social Exclusion Unit was charged with reporting to the Prime Minister on how to 'develop integrated and sustainable approaches to the problems of the worst housing estates, including crime, drugs, unemployment, community breakdown and bad schools'.

The Social Exclusion Unit's remit is to shift the focus of programmes to prevention rather than cure, and to co-ordinate policy better between programmes and government departments. It is an experiment in holistic government and can be seen as an attempt to break down conflict between government departments (McCormick and Leicester 1998). Tackling exclusion is an ongoing process, not an outcome to be achieved by pulling together the appropriate policy levels either at Westminster or in Edinburgh.

The clearest factor in excluding people from the mainstream is poverty. The largest single group below average income is composed of working-age couples and their children, followed by pensioners, and single parents and their children. The true extent of such exclusions is not known, largely due to the fact that sections of the population, such as the homeless, are not included in surveys.

The strongest cause of exclusion is lack of work. Children grow up in poverty because their parents do not have jobs. Pensioners retire in poverty because their earnings were not enough to provide a decent pension (in addition to changes in the state's side of the 'contract' between the generations). The least qualified are significantly more likely to be unemployed. Poor health, disability, care responsibilities, separation and divorce are among the other factors across people's lives which increase the risk of long-term poverty, above all among women. And there is a particularly strong risk of poor educational attainment among children in care (McCormick and Leicester 1998).

Social exclusion is multidimensional and therefore has implications for a wide range of agencies and organisations. The need for holistic 'joined-up' partnerships and multi-agency responses to social exclusion is an important thread. The partnership approach is also intended to open the way for 'policy innovation' to overcome the compartmentalisation of policy issues inside the domains of separate agencies and to facilitate new alliances and ways of understanding and reacting to problems.

In Scotland, the government has developed its own policy in order to deal with social exclusion. It is called *Social Inclusion – Opening the Door to a Better Scotland* (SOHD 1999b). Essentially, social inclusion addresses the same issues that exist in England. The focus of the work in social inclusion is collective action whereby different agencies will work together in order to reduce inequalities. Two themes emerge in this enterprise, that of community development and the concept of empowerment.

Community development

Community development involves working with communities, incorporating the views of ordinary people and voluntary groups in the assessment of needs and the development of appropriate response (Bracht 1999). The first lesson that should guide a strategy for community involvement is to know the history of the area and to look at existing signs of 'embedded' or reactive community activity. What joint activities, networks and organisations already exist on the inhabitants' own initiative? What practical help can they call on? What obstacles do they face? In simple terms, for community development to work to achieve change, a community needs to be aware of their specific needs and to want specific changes. This stimulates people to think about what they might do to bring about such changes by taking action themselves (for more information about the stages of community development see Batten 1967 in Tones and Tilford 1994: 276).

Community development is a tremendous challenge and requires substantial and highly skilled resources. Central to community development is participation. Unlike a topic-based approach to promoting health, participation should be voluntary and owned by the community. It should not be imposed. The key concepts of community development are equity, collective action, participation, collaboration and empowerment. Equity means that communities should have equal access to resources, and this includes services. Collective action involves people grouping together to address problems, providing mutual support and acting together around a common aim to bring about some change they have identified. Participation involves communities in making decisions which will improve their health. Collaboration is working together, sharing resources and skills and empowerment and can be described as the process by which people gain control over their lives.

The benefits of a community development approach to promoting health is that it encourages people to identify what they want, which in turn could help service providers to highlight gaps and overlaps in services. Community development provides a framework and methods for tackling inequalities, and this should lead to achieving more equity. It also promotes community participation, which in itself can increase confidence in attempting to resolve issues around inequalities.

The spectrum of participation (Brager and Specht 1973, cited in Tones and Tilford 1994) offers a valuable perspective on the relationship between participation and power.

Spectrum of participation by member of a community

Level of participation	*Action by participant*
Low	**None**
	- the community is told nothing: therefore participation is impossible
	Receives information
	- the community is told what is planned and compliance is expected
	Is consulted
	- compliance is sought through developing support for the plan
	Advises
	- the nature of the intervention is still top down, but there is sufficient flexibility to allow for the community to suggest changes
	Involved in planning
	- there is a greater expectation of change from the organisers
	Has authority
	- the community are involved in the planning process from the outset, but there's still a top-down element
	Has control
	- the community both identity the problems and
High	seek the solution
	(Brager and Specht 1973, cited in Tones and Tilford 1994)

Many projects that have been established to deal with inequalities in health are only funded for two to three years. During this time it is unlikely that any major change will occur. This is an issue for project leaders who inevitably have to produce a report at the end of the funding period in order to gain further funding. Stakeholders usually require some form of quantitative data to show that the project has met its objectives either wholly or in part. Attempts to reduce health inequality are not always dependent on numbers, but on people's opinions and attitudes towards their health and the health of their community, which is mainly a matter of qualitative judgement.

Dr Elaine Mullen (2000) highlights the problem of evaluating community health promotion. She refers to a community project, the Strides Sexual Health Project that was funded for three years by a health authority in Wales. The purpose of the project was to reduce sexually transmitted infections (STIs) and teenage pregnancies. Funding was conditional on the outcome of an evaluation. Four issues emerged. The project was based on the rationale that, by raising self-esteem, the organisers would empower people and increase the availability of choices and the feeling of control over exercising these choices (Mullen 2000).

It would be considered unrealistic for a three-year project to lead to a decline in teenage pregnancies or STIs. If there were such a decline, it would be difficult to attribute this directly to the project for a variety of reasons. If there is a lack of evidence then the risk of funding being withdrawn becomes a reality. There is a need for stakeholders to adopt different criteria for evidence-based community health promotion.

In Glasgow, tenants on the Greater Easterhouse Estate carried out a long campaign which eventually persuaded the local council to install a more efficient heating system throughout the damp, unhealthy flats. Their success saved tenants thousands of pounds a year in heating bills, more than paid for its cost to the council in savings on repairs, and saved the health authority a lot of expense as well.

The Easterhouse heating campaign was unusual in documenting its economic effects, but it is quite obvious that all such activities must have a considerable economic value (Chanan 2000). If community development is successful then it is likely that individuals and communities will be empowered.

Empowerment

Tones (Tones and Tilford 1994) differentiate between empowerment and participation. He goes on to say that an empowered person is more likely to engage in active community participation than someone who is helplessly apathetic. On the other hand, participation may contribute to empowerment.

Empowerment is the process through which people, organisations and communities gain mastery over their lives. This process includes: acknowledging people as experts in their own health, seeing autonomy and self-determination as health goals, emphasising abilities and building on them, raising the esteem of individuals and communities through valuing their knowledge and experience, supporting people to become competent participants in community activities, promoting confidence by enabling the development of new skills and opportunities, and supporting the emergence of leadership from within the community. Central to the concept of empowerment is the word 'power'. The aim of empowerment is to challenge the power base, therefore returning to individuals the ownership of their own destiny.

During the 1980s the word 'empowerment' became widespread in the field of health promotion and is now considered an essential part of promoting positive health. The concept of empowerment is no longer just part of health promotion. It is part of the vocabulary of other health professionals, such as nurses, physiotherapists, occupational therapists and dieticians, to name but a few. Empowerment has gained recognition over the years in that it encompasses a holistic approach to health. The author has identified evidence which suggests that it is now an integral part of undergraduate programmes in health promotion and is an essential part of the curriculum.

Carey (2000) suggests that empowerment has its roots in liberatory pedagogy; a concept which effectively refers to freedom through education. Carey looked at the work of Paulo Freire, who believed that education was the means by which subordinate groups could challenge the systems behind their oppression and so improve their position in life. The aim of empowerment is to challenge the power base. This will occur if there is a process of 'concientisation', or critical conciousness-raising. Tones (Tones and Tilford 1994) in his model of health education also mentions critical consciousness-raising as one of the steps required in order to influence healthy public policy.

Freire draws the distinction between three forms of human consciousness. He describes these as 'magic', 'naïve' and 'critical' (see Carey 2000). Magic consciousness refers to the attribution of the cause of events to superior powers, such as a deity. This state is essentially fatalistic and implies that the individual has no authority over his or her circumstances. Naïve consciousness constitutes an acknowledgement of the causes of events, but these are accepted uncritically. The individual has some sense of the situation, but no understanding of why it should be challenged, never mind how it could be challenged. The process of concientisation moves us from magic or naïve thinking into a more critical mode of exploring our existence, which involves reflections on reality. The outcome of this process is the identification of the causes of this reality, consideration of their implications and the development of plans to transform reality. The next step from concientisation, and the ultimate aim of empowerment, is 'praxis'. This embraces a constant interaction between action for change and reflection on this action. As a result, the change process is continually subjected to critical reflection. This will ensure that people will embark upon change in an open, honest and discriminating manner.

If this process were applied to present-day practice, then it is more likely that communities would be truly empowered. Although the present government encourages public involvement in developing health services, it is not clear how this can be achieved. It is questionable whether those in power, such as governments, truly want to transfer power to local communities or indeed whether communities should take on the responsibility for decisions in healthcare provision. Another question is whether we actually empower people or only enable them to improve things.

Health improvement

New Labour policies on healthcare, as exemplified by *New NHS: Modern and Dependable* (DoH 1997) and *Designed to Care: Renewing the Health Service in Scotland* (SOHD 1997) concentrated on a better integrated health service. They introduced health improvement plans (HImPs) which are three-year local action plans implemented by the main statutory and voluntary bodies in each Health Authority and Health Board. The purpose of these plans is to encourage agencies to work together to plan and deliver measures to improve the health of the local population (DoH 1997). Therefore, it is essential to establish a collaborative approach between the NHS and other organisations where decisions on community services, housing, employment and the environment can influence health.

A study carried out by the King's Fund showed that there is considerable enthusiasm and goodwill for the concept of health improvement programmes. They were seen as providing opportunities to address the wider determinants of health, tackle inequalities and inequities in access to services, share responsibility for an ambitious and important agenda and develop partnership working (Arora *et al.* 2000).

Saving Lives: Our Healthier Nation (DoH 1999) proposed a national contract between government, local agencies, communities and individuals, each with their own role to play in improving the health of the population as a whole, while also improving the health of the worst off at a faster pace so as to narrow the health gap.

The proposed 'contracts' appeared quite heavily weighted towards local obligations. In relation to social exclusion the use of a 'healthy setting' approach, focusing on schools, workplace and neighbourhoods as vehicles for health improvement, seemed itself to be soundly exclusive (for instances, see Welsh Office 1997, 1998).

NHS bodies and local government authorities have a statutory duty to co-operate in improving health and welfare as well as co-operating in improvement plans for health and healthcare.

While responsibility for public health continues to be retained at Health Authorities and Health Boards levels, the responsibility for health improvement has been devolved to community level and is the responsibility of Primary Care Groups and Local Healthcare Co-operatives. These have been established so that GPs, public health nurses and public health co-ordinators will collaborate with local authorities and other agencies to identify the health needs of local populations and develop plans for health improvement.

French (French and Learmouth 1998) has identified five key factors, which could be used as indicators for Health Improvement Programmes.

Five Key Action Areas	Input/Process
Healthy public policy	Advocacy for local policies that promote health
Improvements in social capital[1]	Comprehensive community development strategy in place
Increase in public participation	Systems developed to allow public to influence decisions
Development of health partnerships	Increasing the percentage of agencies and businesses which are involved in health alliance work
A healthier environment	Air quality measurement systems in place

Note

[1] The term 'social capital' has come to play an increasingly important role in contemporary debate about the structure and development of modern society and in particular the related problems of the democratic deficit and social exclusion. See Alcock and Mason (2001).

Government guidance on health improvement programmes published in 1998 required that they should:

- set a strategic framework for action on national and local priorities, setting targets and milestones for measurable improvement;
- include needs assessment and resource mapping;
- include local joint investment plans and a service and financial framework;
- include an account of the nature and extent of past and future involvement of the stakeholders in preparing the HImP;
- be made available widely in accessible forms.

In essence, these guidelines are open to interpretation, which means that individual health authorities and health boards can adapt them to meet the needs of local people. On a positive note, the guidelines allow for a strategic approach to health improvement of local populations, which can be evaluated.

In 1990 the NHS and Community Care Act stated that regional health authorities and local authorities were required to assess health and social needs as a means of obtaining accurate and appropriate information on which to base policy. (Hawtin *et al.* 1994).

Needs assessment is a tool used to identify priority areas and to allocate resources accordingly. However, it should be recognised that any needs assessment, which involves the local population, runs the risk of raising expectations. These expectations may not be met for a variety of reasons, which includes resources constraints.

The other main issues relating to the guidelines is that of interagency working. This would depend entirely on how different stakeholders have worked together in the past and how each of the stakeholders involved perceives the concept of health improvement.

Abbott and Gillan (2000) scrutinised a sample of 36 HImPs. The purpose of this was to look for evidence of local commitment to:

- national and local priorities for health improvement
- public consultation
- partnership working
- a strategy driven by identified health needs
- effective implementation of the strategy

The total number of priorities set was 457, a mean of 13 per HImP. Twelve HImPs have between 6 and 10 priorities, 17 had between 11 and 20, and five had more than 20. The highest number of priorities was 28. It was interesting to note that only 9 HImPs identified social determinants of health as a priority. Given that HImPs are supposed to address inequalities, this is a rather low number. Twenty-nine of the HImPs analysed recorded some consultation with the public, including the following representative groups and organisations: Community Health Councils (23); local health-related groups (19); carer groups (13) and other community groups (20)

A key aspect of HImPs is that health authorities should have consulted widely with local partnership agencies in drawing these up, and that such agencies should be committed to delivering the programmes. Most (33) mentioned a range of partner organisations. Thirteen simply provided a list, whereas the remainder (20) gave some indication of the roles and responsibilities that partner agencies had agreed to take on. Most HImPs gave details of other joint working with local authorities (29) or with local NHS Trusts (22) and referred to other local strategic planning documents in some detail (26). Nineteen referred to the joint investment plans drawn up with local authorities. About half of the HImPs (19) met PCGs priorities. Only nine included details of PCGs primary care investment plans. A search for evidence on how the priorities would be delivered was carried out. Health authorities were required to refer to service and financial frameworks in the HImP: 29 did so fully, 20 in some detail and 9 only briefly. A search for evidence relating to monitoring and performance was also carried out. Only 7 HImPs included any measurable targets. Other HImPs had milestones such as a working group to report by April 2000.

Wistow (2000) comments on the new White Paper on health service provision and states that 'health services, however modern and dependable, are only one of the determinants of health at individual and collective levels'. He adds: 'the wider modernisation agenda supported this understanding of public health. It advocated "joined up" government to tackle the causes of poverty and social exclusion, not just the symptoms.'

Healthy alliances – interagency working

Sue Jelly (2001) stated that tackling inequalities in health requires an integrated approach with everyone pulling together. This suggests that if we are to reduce inequalities then there needs to be successful interagency working. She goes on to say that health professionals must find effective ways of working with communities – and all agencies must take account of the kind of support local people need to participate in local initiatives. The concept of interagency working was first introduced by the government in 1992 in its health strategy *The Health of the Nation* (DoH 1992). Interagency working requires collaboration between agencies in order to meet the needs of local populations.

The National Health Service (NHS) and local authorities (LAs) have a mandate for interagency working, but for interagency working to be successful, other agencies such as voluntary bodies need to be involved. Involvement of these agencies is often based on goodwill or a commitment to improving the health of local populations by the process of social inclusion.

Just because health authorities and health boards initiate interagency working, it does not always follow that they will take the lead. It is important to recognise that all agencies involved in interagency working have ownership of the work undertaken and therefore the most appropriate leader should be chosen.

Douglas (1998) produced an extended framework for assessing the potential performance and achievement of healthy alliances. There are three broad areas: assessing potential, joint working and assessing achievements. Assessing potential allows for an analysis of past and present relationships. This is important so that any conflict can be identified and dealt with. The core purpose and priorities of each of the agencies involved need to be clarified in order to examine areas of similarity and overlap. The nature and extent of the planned collaboration in some way is a result of an analysis of the other two.

For joint working to be a success, several issues need to be addressed. These include resource exchange, user involvement, leadership and co-ordinated activity. Resource exchange between agencies is sometimes recognised as a barrier to interagency working. For example the NHS and LAs have their own budgets which often raises questions such as who is responsible for delivery and who provides the finance. This needs to be addressed once the collaboration is identified. The second issue to address is that of user involvement. Who decides which member of the community will be involved in the planning of an initiative? Will the person chosen be representative of the community? This can often lead to conflict because of possible hidden agendas. If selection is based on community development, then it is more likely to produce a successful collaboration. The third issue to be addressed is leadership style. If the leader of the initiative is too authoritarian then the collaboration is likely to fail. The process of decision making needs to be a democratic process, which will ultimately lead to ownership of the initiative. However, the leader needs to be skilled in order to guide the agencies towards a collaboration which is going to be successful. The final area needing to be addressed is that of assessing achievements or evaluation of the initiative. The debate here is whether this assessment or evaluation is quantitative or qualitative. It should be recognised that, historically, a quantitative approach to assessment or evaluation is preferred by the stakeholders, simply because any change can be seen in numerical terms. However, the outcomes of successful interagency working cannot always be quantified, encouraging the view that qualitative data should be recognised as being just as important and valid. The final issue to be addressed is the extent to which organisational learning takes place through interagency working.

For interagency working to be successful there is a need for a greater under-standing of how different agencies are structured and how they operate. Furthermore, each agency has its own culture. Therefore it is important that those co-ordinating interagency working are aware of these cultures and how they may be in conflict. If conflict exists between cultures, then it is unlikely that there will successful outcomes. For this reason, every attempt to resist conflict should be made to ensure that there is equity across cultures.

A familiar term used in public services is multidisciplinary or interdisciplinary team working. Woodcock and Francis (1989) provide a definition of a 'team', namely: 'a group of people who share common objectives and who need to work together to achieve them'. A multidisciplinary team is a team of professionals working together for the benefit of the patient/client but retaining their professional autonomy. Interdisciplinary teams, on the other hand, are teams which work as a collective for the benefit of the patient/client. This means that an interdisciplinary team shares responsibility and resources and is not focused on retaining professional autonomy. Applied to interagency working, the principles are the same with the local population at the centre. Agencies need to work as a team in order to achieve a common goal. For teams to be successful, members need to give up some of their professional autonomy. For some this may be difficult and attempts to retain professional autonomy continue to dominate.

Alliances or interagency working tend to be made up of multidisciplinary organisational representatives which operate within specialised environments and which may offer harmonious, alien, conflicting and/or stimulating communication systems within which to develop agendas, organise tasks and agree monitoring and evaluation strategies. All of this implies that there need to be equal partnerships while retaining truthfulness.

One of the main characteristics of interagency working is the building of trust between different agencies. It could be that an imbalance between organisations could lead to competition, which inhibits successful interagency working. The purpose of the government's White Paper *Designed to Care: Renewing the Health Service* was to eliminate competition and introduce co-operation (SOHD 1997). Agencies therefore need to develop their own culture, which would result in co-operation, which, in turn, would lead to successful working for the benefit of the local population.

For interagency working to be successful, it requires a long-term approach together with appropriate funding and resources. Interagency working should, of course, be based on people and their organisational relationships. These are determined by interactions among goals and objectives, structure, style of leadership and the behaviour of people. This is described by Mullins (1998) as 'organisational climate'. He identified thirteen different characteristics, which need to be in place for an organisational climate to be healthy. The following relate to interagency working such as:

- integrational goals and personal goals;
- democratic functioning of the organisation with full opportunities for participation; mutual trust, consideration and support among different levels of the organisation;
- open discussion of conflict with an attempt to avoid confrontation;
- managerial behaviour and styles of leadership appropriate to the particular work situation;
- recognition of peoples' needs and expectations at work, and individual differences at attributes;
- a sense of identity with, and loyalty to, the organisation and feeling of being a valued and important member.

For those involved in interagency working, there needs to be a commitment to achieving goals and objectives. White, cited by Mullins (1998), suggests three kinds of behaviours, which denote 'commitment' to the organisation in which a person works:

- belief in, and acceptance of the organisation itself and/or its goals and values;
- willingness to exert effort on behalf of the organisation about the contract of employment;
- desire to remain with the organisation.

Commitment is also always voluntary and personal. It cannot be imposed, others cannot initiate it, and it can be withdrawn.

For interagency working to be successful, every effort should be made to build a true team. Individual members should contribute to a common goal.

If this does not happen then there is likelihood that there will be friction, frustration and conflict. Conflict is based on the incompatibility of goals and arises in opposing behaviours, for example, conflict situations. However, conflict should not always be seen in negative terms. Some of the positive aspects of conflict are the production of better ideas; people are forced to search for new approaches; long-standing problems are often brought to the surface and resolved through clarification of individual views; stimulation of interest and creativity; a chance for people to test their capacities (Schmidt 1974, cited in Mullins 1998), all can take place.

The negative aspects of conflict include some people feeling defeated and demeaned; the distance between people is increased; a climate of mistrust and suspicion is developed; individuals and groups concentrate on their own narrow interests; and resistance is developed, rather that teamwork.

There are many sources of possible conflict in interagency working. For example, individuals within each agency may have different perceptions, whereby they see things in a different way, which could lead to a lack of co-operation. Each agency will have its own budget and resources. Therefore, to reduce this possible source of conflict there needs to be equity of distribution. It may be that there is a lack of joined-up working whereby the work of one agency is dependent on the work of another. Therefore, to reduce conflict, each agency needs to have a common goal towards which they are working. This requires that clear role definitions should be established. It is possible that each agency is protective of its own autonomy and does not welcome interference from other organisations. Other possible sources of conflict are environmental changes, such as government interventions, a shift in demand or social values. All of these possible sources should be addressed in order to eliminate conflict. If conflict does exist in interagency work, it can be overcome by clarifying the goals and objectives, resource distribution, the development of interpersonal and group processes, and by an increase in group activity, and a more supportive leadership style.

Mullins (1998) describes public sector organisations as being owned by the general public and financed by government through central and local funding. He goes on to say that public sector organisations do not distribute profits and the main aim is a service to and for the well-being of the community (Mullins, 1998).

Organisational culture

For some, interagency working will be a challenge because traditionally they have often worked in isolation. Through working in isolation it is likely that each agency will develop their own culture. What we mean by 'culture' is a set of artefacts, beliefs, values, norms and ground rules which significantly influences how the agency will operate (Beckhard and Harris 1987; for more on these, see Mullins 1998). Therefore, for agencies to work together successfully, they need to know and understand each other's culture.

Handy describes four main types of organisation culture: power culture; role culture; task culture; and person culture (Handy, 1993). Power culture is dependent on a central power source, which may be a central figure in the organisation. This person is likely to have complete control, which would affect the way that individuals within the organisation will work together. There is the likelihood that there will be no ground rules on which to base trust and empathy between the workforce. Power cultures are potentially destructive in that the working team will not have ownership of the work in hand. Lack of ownership by the workforce could lead to working in isolation and to the failure of interagency working.

Role culture is often stereotyped as a bureaucracy and is hierarchical. In this situation position power is the main source of power. This hierarchy is made up of specialists or people in senior management positions. For example, the National Health Service is made up of professions such as medicine, nursing, professions allied to medicine and management, each of which has their own culture. This is often referred to as 'tribalism' and the profession or job description becomes more important than the individual. The chief executive or the consultant normally holds position power.

Task culture is job- or project-oriented. Task culture seeks to bring together the right resources and people who work as a team and have a common goal. By having a task culture, influence is widely distributed, which reduces hierarchy. Each individual is perceived as an expert and contributes equally to the business of the organisation. Task culture is based on teamwork and not on position or personal power.

Person culture sees the individual as the central focus and any structure exists to service the individuals within it. Groups of people will come together and recognise that working together is in their own interest. The National Health Service could be criticised for not having a person culture because is too bureaucratic and hierarchical. Person culture occurs if there is mutual consent by individuals, which means that they work together because they want to. This way of working could be likened to an interdisciplinary team whereby a group of professionals come together and work together for the benefit of the patient and their carers. Individuals have almost complete autonomy and any influence over them is likely to be on the basis of personal power.

In order to address differing cultural issues, organisational learning needs to take place. Organisations can only become effective if the people selected to run them are capable of two key skills – learning continuously and giving direction (Garratt 1987). Learning continuously involves taking time out to think and learn about different organisations. This may result in feelings of frustration because to take time out to think means that there is less time to do the job. In addition, there may be opposition to this type of approach because people are too busy dealing with the day-to-day business of the organisations. It may be that there are no mechanisms for open debate and refining policy and strategy on a given project, in which case protected time needs to be built in at the planning stage. How well any organisation can do depends on factors such as internal communication and the assimilation of individual knowledge into new work structures, routines and norms. However, learning is not always about acquisition. There is also a need for learning strategies that focus on 'unlearning' previously established ways of doing things. The organisation should develop the ability to identify, evaluate and change whole routines embedded in organisational custom (Davis and Nutley 2000). Senge (cited in Davies and Nutley 2000), provides key features of a learning organisation.

Key features of a learning organisation

Open systems thinking Individuals within organisations can tend to see activities in an isolated way, disconnected from the whole. Open systems thinking encapsulates the notion of teaching people to reintegrate activities, to see how what they do and what others do are interconnected. This reintegration needs to stretch beyond internal departmental boundaries, and even beyond the boundaries of the organisation itself, to encompass other services.

Improving individual capabilities For an organisation to be striving for excellence,the individuals within that organisation must constantly be improving their own personal proficiencies.

Team learning Team learning is vital because it is largely through teams that organisations achieve their objectives. Development of the whole team rather than individual learning is essential.

Updating mental models Mental models' are the deeply held assumptions and generalisations formed by individuals (internally and often implicitly). These models influence how people make sense of the world. They control, for example, how causes and effects are linked conceptually and constrain what individuals see as possible within the organisation. Changing and updating these mental models is essential to finding new ways of doing things

A cohesive vision   Empowering and enabling individuals within an organisation has to be counterbalanced by providing clear strategic direction and articulating a coherent set of values that can guide individual actions. Encouraging a shared understanding of this vision and commitment to it is crucial in building a learning organisation

Adapted from Senge (in Davies and Nutley 2000).

If these key features are applied to interagency working, then it is likely that organisational culture issues will be addressed which will lead to success.

Conclusion

Since health inequalities were first identified in the 1980s, health promotion has seen this as a challenge. The government of the day refused to accept that the health of the population was not only affected by lifestyle factors, but also affected by social factors such as poverty, unemployment, bad housing, poor education and working conditions. In addition, a number of sections of the community were socially excluded from our society. This included the elderly, the disabled, people with HIV/AIDS, drug abusers, people with mental illness, ethnic minorities and the homeless, to name but a few. This left health promotion departments in something of a dilemma. Should they focus on the physical and lifestyle aspects of health, such as smoking, healthy eating, exercise, sexually transmitted infections, dental health, as they did in the days of health education, or should they attempt to tackle the wider determinants of health?

Community development and empowerment emerged as an important field of operation in health promotion in the 1980s. This may have been seen in simplistic terms and not seen as a long-term investment in health. Many community development and empowerment projects were set up over the years. At best they attracted short-term funding for a maximum of three years, hardly enough time to address the issues that are associated with health inequalities. These issues could not be dealt with in any depth. Community development and empowerment projects take time to develop into something meaningful. They should be owned and developed by the community or individuals and not by the individual employed as a project worker. Community development and empowerment requires sustainability for it to be successful. Short-term projects which come to an end are likely to leave communities and individuals with a feeling of frustration that their work has not been recognised, or feelings of mistrust of stakeholders whose expectations of community development and empowerment may be unrealistic. The evaluation of community development and empowerment is intrinsically difficult because they do not involve tangible concepts, unlike lifestyle, which is quantifiable. The success of community development and empowerment projects can be seen in terms of a change in attitudes, opinions and skills of the community and individuals they are designed to help.

Government policies of the early 1990s did not address health inequalities. Documents only briefly referred to health inequalities or 'health variation'. The focus of these documents was on lifestyle factors such as smoking, exercise, nutrition, dental health, drugs and HIV/AIDS. Unlike community development and empowerment these 'topics' lend themselves to high-profile health promotion activities which, at best, will only raise awareness of the general population. They will not change behaviour. These topics are linked to the major causes of mortality and morbidity in the United Kingdom, which can be measured by those in power. Any reduction in mortality and morbidity would be welcomed by the government and wrongly attributed to high-profile health promotion. The focus on topics meant that community development and empowerment became less attractive to stakeholders because of the time commitment that would be required, or because they would not necessarily produce tangible results.

With the New Labour government, there was a renewed interest in reducing health inequalities. The government introduced health improvement plans, which are three-year plans designed to address health inequalities. The purpose of those plans was to encourage interagency or 'joined-up' working which would result in an improvement in the health of local populations. Along with health improvement plans came social inclusion partnerships. The underlying philosophy of the social inclusion partnerships is the same: that different agencies would work together to address the issues associated with health inequalities. However, there is still an issue about the sustainability of these partnerships, given that they come with a time limit.

Interagency working requires that each agency involved understands how the others are structured and operate. Each agency will have its own discrete culture and it may be that these cultures will be in conflict with each other. If conflict exists, then it is likely that the outcome will be unsuccessful. Conflict, however, should not always be seen in negative terms. Some of the positive aspects of conflict are the production of better ideas. People have the opportunity to increase dialogue in order to search for new solutions to a particular problem. 'It is good to talk.' There is also the opportunity for long-standing problems to be brought to the surface, allowing clarification and respect for individual views and opinions. If this process were encouraged then 'joined-up' working and increase in trust would ensue.

Finally, if health inequalities are to be addressed, agencies need to understand different organisational cultures, which exist and work as a team to achieve a common goal. Every attempt should be made to eliminate hidden agendas.

References

Abbott, S. and Gillam, S. (2000) 'Trusting to Luck', *Health Service Journal* 110(5705): 24–5.

Acheson, Sir D. (1998) *Public Health in England: The Report of the Committee of Inquiry into the Future Development of the Public Health Function*, Cm 289. London: HMSO.

Alcock, P. and Mason, P. (2001) 'Should We Invest in Social Capital?', *Department of Social Work: Working Paper*. Birmingham: University of Birmingham.

Arora, S., Davies, A. and Thomson, S. (2000) 'Developing Health Improvement Programmes: Challenges for the New Millennium', *Journal of Interprofessional Care* 14(1): 9–18.

Beckhard, R. and Harris, R.T. (1987) *Organisational Transitions*, 2nd edn. Wokingham: Addison-Wesley Publishing Company.

Benzeval, M., Dilnot, A., Judge, K. and Taylor, J. (2000) 'Income and Health over the Lifecourse: Evidence and Policy Implications', in H. Graham (ed.) *Understanding Health Inequalities*. Buckingham: Open University Press.

Black, D. (1988) *The Black Report*, in N. Davidson and P. Townsend, (eds) *Inequalities in Health*. London: Penguin.

Bracht, N. (ed.) (1999) *Health Promotion at the Community Level: New Advances*. London: Sage.

Brager, C. and Specht, H. (1973) *Community Organising*. Columbia: Columbia University Press.

Bunton, R. and McDonald, G. (1992) *Health Promotion: Disciplines and Diversity*. London: Routledge.

Carey, P. (2000) 'Community Health and Empowerment', in J. Kerr (ed.) *Community Health Promotion: Challenges for Practice*. London: Bailliere Tindall.

Chanan, G. (2000) 'Community Responses to Social Exclusion', in J. Percy-Smith (ed.) *Policy Responses to Social Exclusion*. Buckingham: Open University Press.

Commission of the European Communities (1993) *Background Report: Social Exclusion – Poverty and Other Social Problems in the European Community*, 1SEC/B11/93. Luxembourg: Office for Official Publications of the European Communities.

Dahlgren, G. and Whitehead, M. (1991) *Policies and Strategies to Promote Social Equity in Health*. Stockholm: Institute for Future Studies.

Davies, H. and Nutley, S. (2000) 'Developing Learning Organisations in the New NHS', *British Medical Journal* 320(7127): 998–1001.

Department of Health (1992) *Health of a Nation*. London: HMSO.

Department of Health (1997) *New NHS: Modern and Dependable*. London: HMSO.

Department of Health (1999) *Saving Lives: Our Healthier Nation*. London: HMSO.

Douglas, R. 'A Framework for Healthy Alliances', in A. Scriven (ed.) *Alliances in Health Promotion*. London: Macmillan.

French, J. (1999) 'Public Health/Health Promotion/Health Development?', *Public Health Forum* 3(3): 718.

French, J. and Learmonth, A. (1998) *Health Improvement Programmes – The Role of Health Promotion Services and the Application of a Social Model of Health to Guide the Process*. Glasgow: Society of Health Education and Health Promotion Specialists.

Garratt, B. (1987) *The Learning Organisation*. Aldershot, Hants: Gower.

Goldblatt, P. and Whitehead, M. (2000) 'Inequalities in Health – Development and Change', *Population Trends* 100: 14–19.

Handy, C.B. (1993) *Understanding Organisations*, 4th edn. London: Penguin.

Hawtin, M., Hughes, G., Percy-Smith, J. and Foreman, A. (1994) *Community Profiling: Auditing Social Needs*. Milton Keynes: Open University Press.

Jelly, S. (2001) 'Editorial', *Health Development Today*. London: Health Development Agency.

McCormick, J. and Leicester, G. (1998) 'Three Nations: Social Exclusion in Scotland', *SCF Paper 3*. Edinburgh: Scottish Council Foundation.

Mullen, E. (2000) 'Hitting the Targets', *Promoting Health* 10: 28–30.

Mullins, L.J. (1996) *Management and Organisation Behaviour* 4th edn. London: Pitman Publishing.

Percy-Smith, J. (ed.) (2000) *Policy Responses to Social Exclusion: Towards Inclusion*. Buckingham: Open University Press.

Scottish Office Health Department (1992) *Scotland's Health: A Challenge to Us All*. Edinburgh: HMSO.

Scottish Office Health Department (1997) *Designed to Care: Renewing the Health Service*. Edinburgh: HMSO.

Scottish Office Health Department (1999a) *Towards a Healthier Scotland*. Edinburgh: HMSO.

Scottish Office Health Department (1999b) *Social Inclusion – Opening the Door to a Better Scotland*. Edinburgh: HMSO.

Schmidt, W.H. (1974) 'Conflict: A Powerful Process for (Good or Bad) Change', *Management Review* 63: 4–10.

Tones, K. and Tilford, S. (1994) *Health Education: Effectiveness, Efficiency and Equity*. London: Chapman Hall.

Welsh Office (1997) *NHS Wales, Putting Patients First*. Cardiff: The Stationery Office.

Welsh Office (1998) *Better Health, Better Wales*. Cardiff: The Stationery Office.

Whitehead, M. (1988) 'The Health Divide', in N. Davidson and P. Townsend (ed.) *Inequalities in Health*. London: Penguin.

WHO (1986) *The Ottawa Charter for Health Promotion*. Geneva: World Health Organization.

WHO (1998) *World Health Organization, Health Promotion Glossary*, HPR/HEP/ 98.1. Geneva: WHO.

Wistow, G. (2000) 'Exclusive Offer?', *Health Service Journal* 110(5727): 26–7.

Woodcock, M. and Francis, D. (1989) *Team Development Manual*. Aldershot: Gower.

Chapter 6

Promoting children's mental health

Developmental and ecological approaches to intervention

Karen Baistow

There are good reasons for paying attention to the mental health of children. The well-documented increase in the rates of mental health problems among children and adolescents in the latter part of the twentieth century has been associated with a heavy personal price paid by them and their families, and significant social and economic costs to their communities. These problems have an impact beyond the clinic and have become a cause for social concern, with salience for us all.

The latter years of the twentieth century saw an increasing awareness, nationally and internationally, of the value of improving the mental health of children. In 1977, for example, a WHO expert committee on child mental health and psychosocial development recommended that governments should be encouraged to formulate policies to promote children's mental health and development (WHO 1977). An important part of the recommendation was that policies should be devised with the involvement, not only of health services, but also of juvenile justice, education and social welfare. More recently, Article 24 of the 1989 United Nations' Convention on Children's Rights stated clearly that children and young people under 18 have the right to 'enjoy the highest attainable standards of [mental] health'. At the beginning of the twenty-first century, the global significance of promoting mental health was confirmed by the World Health Organization, which identified the prevention of mental disorders and the promotion of mental health as one of its priority projects under the *Mental Health Global Action Programme* (WHO 2002: 4). This rise in interest has, in part, come about as a result of gradual successes in combating preventable child mortality during the twentieth century, and associated efforts to enhance the health and development of those children who survived infancy (Graham and Orley 1998; Meyers 1992). Over the last hundred years, notions of health have broadened, and the focus on children has widened to include their psychological, social and emotional, as well as physical development (Baistow 1995, 2001; Costello and Angold 2000). A corollary of this interest in psychosocial health and development is a recognition of maladjustment and mental health problems, and their effects on individuals, families and communities. The increasing incidence of troubled and troublesome children both reflects and shapes this recognition, and public concern is growing about the personal and social impact of their difficulties. These children's problems cover a range of psychological difficulties, in which there may be disturbances in functioning of mood, relationships, behaviour or development. They often involve considerable distress. It is important to remember that, as well as those children with diagnosed psychiatric disorders, there are much larger numbers of children, who, though falling below the threshold of formal diagnosis, also warrant special attention because their behaviour causes significant concern and disruption to themselves, their families and communities.

Evidence is accumulating of the serious emotional, social and economic costs that are associated with increasing rates of mental health problems in children and young people and, as significantly, of the benefits to children, their families and their communities that can result from prevention efforts and mental health promotion (McGuire and Earls 1991). This chapter examines the evidence and considers the implications for the development of mental health promotion approaches that take into account the role of 'community' for mental health and the vital importance of children's mental health for community. It is divided into four parts. The first section offers a rationale for mental health promotion by describing the scale and extent of childhood mental health problems and their impact on the child, the family and the community. Section two considers risk and resilience, examining the causes of children's mental health (problems) in terms of multi-factorial and interconnected processes of risk and resilience. This position is not only theoretically attractive; as we will see, while it has implications for our *understanding* of treatment, care, prevention and promotion, it can also provide a sound basis for *intervention* efforts. This section provides an overview of evidence that certain factors at the levels of individual, family and community are associated with increased vulnerability to mental health problems, while others appear to protect the individual and promote resilience in the face of adversity. The implications for prevention and mental health promotion are discussed in the third section, which draws on the previous two sections to emphasise the value of adopting an ecological approach, seeing 'the child' and 'childhood' in their social and developmental contexts. Using examples from different continents, this final section considers a range of interventions, including those that target mental health issues directly and other approaches which seek to promote mental health by enhancing the ecologies of the child, the family and the community.

The rationale for promoting children's mental health

One of the most powerful arguments for promoting children's mental health lies in the scale of the problem. National and international surveys report prevalence rates at about 15–20 per cent (Audit Commission 1999; Brandenburg *et al.* 1990; Mental Health Foundation 1999; Offord *et al.* 1987). This means that, at any one time, about one in five children and adolescents (from pre-school to 20 years) suffers from mental health problems. These problems range from emotional disorders such as anxiety and depression (12 per cent) and conduct disorders (10 per cent), to less common but more intractable disorders such as autism, affecting less than 1 per cent of children. There are also indications that there are considerable numbers of troubled children who, though not meeting standardised diagnostic criteria, nevertheless experience substantial distress, or behave in ways that are significantly troublesome (e.g. Clarke *et al.* 1997, cited in Macdonald and Bower 2000). Studies agree that these rates, which are common to many industrialised countries, represent a substantial increase since the end of the Second World War and numbers of recorded problems continue to rise. In addition, many of these children will experience a number of difficulties at the same time. In the recent Audit Commission report into child and adolescent health services in England and Wales *Children in Mind* (1999), fewer than 5 per cent of children attending these services presented with only one problem, while 16 per cent had five and nearly 10 per cent had eight presenting problems. The types of problem that presented most frequently were family life and relationships, problems involving emotional and related symptoms, peer relationships and disruptive, anti-social or aggressive behaviour. If we focus on particular categories of children, a further cause for concern arises, where it becomes clear that, as with adult mental illness, children's mental health problems are not equally distributed in the population. Thus there are higher proportions of children with these problems among, for example, those who live in materially disad-vantaged circumstances (Bradley and Corwyn 2002; Brooks-Gunn and Duncan 1997; Meltzer *et al.* 2000), among young offenders (Rutter *et al.* 1998), those who are in the care of local authorities (McCann 1996) and those who are the children of lone parents (McMunn *et al* 2001; Meltzer *et al.* 2000). As we will see in the discussion of risk in the section below, living in these circumstances and, for many children, experiencing more than one form of adversity, can pose substantial threats to their well-being, both in the short and long term.

This brings us to the second reason for paying attention to children's mental health: the connections between mental health problems and a range of other disadvantaging difficulties which together can profoundly affect the life chances of children, their families, and the stability and cohesion of communities. The connections between child and adolescent mental health problems, and a range of behaviours that are the cause of growing public concern – including, juvenile crime, drug and alcohol misuse, self-harm and eating disorders (Rutter and Smith 1995) – suggest that if we are to develop mental health promotion strategies that really make a difference, we need to broaden our notions of child welfare and the conditions which foster it.

One of the most important associations, which has ramifications for individuals and communities, is between mental health and educational problems. This has been well documented, in terms of the overlap of risk factors for both low educational attainment and anti-social behaviour in school. Children with learning difficulties, either because of low IQ or a specific learning disorder, are at increased risk of mental health problems (Graham 1985), and those with mental health problems are much more likely to have special educational needs (Meltzer *et al.* 2000). Emotional and behavioural problems have educational and social repercussions on the school as the 'containing' community, especially in terms of the disruptive effects on pupils and teachers, classroom functioning and school-wide morale. Behavioural problems have been found to be the most common reason for school exclusions in the UK (Barnes 1998). While excluding children with emotional and behavioural problems can help schools, there are personal and social costs associated with this increasing trend (Barnes 1998; Hayden 1994; Parsons 1996). For the already vulnerable child or young person, school exclusion often means exposure to circumstances and behaviours which pose further risks to their mental health. The wider community into which they are expelled becomes a key site of their problem behaviours, but, without the resources to cope, as is the case in many parts of the UK, community responses to these children have shifted in recent years away from therapeutic and educational approaches towards a criminal justice model. As we noted above, the rate of mental health problems is high in young offenders, particularly persistent offenders, and the risk factors for youth crime include not only mental health problems but also substance misuse and teenage pregnancy as well as school failure (Rutter *et al.* 1998). For those who remain in school, the effects of the interplay between educational and mental health difficulties extend beyond the school years into a high risk of further mental health problems (Barnes 1998), low employability and reduced job opportunities, and an increased likelihood of problematic relationships and social isolation (Kurtz 1996). The coexistence of these problem behaviours represents a multiple and compound risk to the future health and welfare of these young people as individuals, spouses and parents. It also negatively affects their potential as citizens and increases the likelihood of their social exclusion.

The links between childhood mental health problems and adult mental illness are a particular cause for concern. A significant number of severe problems in childhood, if not adequately treated, lead to enduring mental illness in adulthood (Target and Fonagy 1996). Though the pathways are not clear, and likely to be multi-factorial, there is mounting evidence that mental health problems in childhood and adolescence, such as depression and conduct disorder, have a poor prognosis and are associated with subsequent co-morbidity with a range of anti-social behaviours (Beardslee *et al.* 1996; Harrington *et al.* 1990; Hofstra *et al.* 2000), increased risks of delinquency as the child grows up and of criminal activity in adulthood (Babinski *et al.* 1999; Farrington *et al.* 1996).

The personal costs of these combined problems, in terms of alienation, distress, under-achievement and social isolation threaten personal well-being. They also affect the health and cohesion of families and communities. Lifelong mental health problems have a pervasive negative impact on individuals' ability to make long-lasting and meaningful social relationships and to belong to supportive social networks. They also diminish the capacity to sustain paid employment. This is a critical factor because, in addition to an income, work contributes to our social role and identity, offers opportunities for new social relationships and brings a structure to our everyday lives. The financial costs of mental illness begin in childhood. The treatment and care of children with mental health problems is expensive for families and communities. However, as these problems are frequently associated with others that also warrant attention, demands are placed not only on health services but also on personal social services, education and juvenile justice services. In a study of conduct disorder in the UK, it emerged that the greatest costs of such children fall on families (37 per cent), schools and their education authority (36 per cent) (Knapp et al. 1999). Findings from a study of the lifetime costs of conduct disorder up to age 28, found that those individuals who had the disorder at the age of 10, cost £100,000 (ten times more) in services than those who did not (Scott et al. 2001). Persisting mental health and social problems mean that, as these children grow older, at the same time as accruing wide ranging costs to their communities, they are also less able to contribute economically to those communities. Low educational attainment and mental health problems are connected with both reduced job opportunities for the individual and a reduced likelihood of a well-educated labour force. Unemployment is bad for our personal health and well-being, and affects the economic and social health of communities. In a demographic context of proportionately more elderly people and fewer young people in the populations of industrialised countries, a healthy and productive workforce becomes a social and economic priority. At a global community level, the WHO, in its *Global Burden of Disease* study, has predicted that by the year 2020, uni-polar major depression will be the second highest cause of disability-adjusted life-years across the world, after ischaemic heart disease, and ahead of road traffic accidents and respiratory diseases (see Murray and Lopez 1997: 1498). Children, as future workers and carers, will therefore be an increasingly valuable resource and one that communities need to collectively nurture to the benefit of all.

Risk and resilience

There is an increasing consensus among policy makers, researchers and those who work in the field, that the first step towards fostering better mental health and well-being among children and young people is to identify those aspects of their lives which put them at risk, and those which offer some protection and promote resilience in the face of difficulties (Department of Health [DoH] 1998; Mental Health Foundation [MHF] 1999). In this section we consider some of the factors that have been found to be associated with risk and resilience.

Studies in the USA and Europe, including the UK, show that a range of factors in children's early lives are consistently associated with increased risks of problems in adolescence and adulthood and, that there is considerable overlap between risk factors for later mental health problems, poor educational outcomes and anti-social behaviour. The risk factors identified for youth crime, for example, have been found to overlap with hard drug use, school age pregnancy, school failure and mental health problems (Rutter *et al.* 1998). Further, risk factors rarely exist on their own and many children are faced during the course of their childhood with a range of difficult circumstances whose impact is both cumulative and compound.

The risks for developing mental health problems in childhood are well documented: for some conditions like autism they are primarily biogenetic but for many others, including emotional and conduct problems, environmental, especially familial factors are implicated. However, though certain risk factors emerge consistently in studies, it is likely that mental health problems in childhood and adolescence arise from an interaction of risks and vulnerabilities rather than simple exposure to risk factors. There is increasing evidence that the presence of risk factors is not in itself sufficient to produce mental health problems; studies show that some children benefit from a range of protective factors which enable them to be resilient, even in the face of very difficult circumstances. Indeed, as we will see later, learning from resilient children and adolescents is becoming an important feature of new developments in prevention and mental health promotion.

Over the last decade there has been a renewed interest in the developmental features of mental health problems, especially focusing on early life and the importance of developmental age and stage in determining how risk factors impact on the child. Since the early post-war years of object-relations theory and the influential work of Bowlby and Winnicott among others, the importance of early mother–child relationships to later development has been the contested subject of psychological, sociological and feminist debates. While debates continue in some quarters, there is an emerging consensus from researchers and clinicians in the fields of child development and psychopathology that parental, especially maternal, responsiveness and attachment are central to development in early infancy, affecting the developing child's ability to learn and their capacity to regulate emotions. Insecure attachment and insensitive and inconsistent care-taking can have powerful and potentially long-lasting effects on the mental health of the developing child (Child Psychotherapy Trust 1999; Crittenden 1995). Further, recent evidence indicates that severe attachment problems, under-stimulation and parental insensitivity can have not only persistent psychological effects but also neurological ones, affecting early brain development and increasing risk for some forms of child psychopathology, (Dawson *et al.* 2000). As well as this focus on the critical importance of infancy and the effects of very early risk factors on later maladjustment, there is increasing attention being paid to evidence from the field of developmental psychopathology which demonstrates the developmental connections between infancy, childhood, adolescence and adulthood. The potential for subsequent experiences to reinforce or to interrupt chains of risk, points to the importance of interventions that are developmentally tailored. Recognising future, as well as current effects of interventions, enhances the possibilities of simultaneously addressing treatment, prevention and mental health promotion (see, for example, Beardslee *et al.* 1996; Cicchetti and Toth 1992; Costello *et al.* 1999; Luthar and Cicchetti 2000).

Risk factors for childhood mental health problems

Epidemiological studies and clinical research point clearly to a powerful association between mental health problems in childhood and adolescence and a constellation of factors which connect parent and child characteristics, parental relationships, family structure and functioning, and social and economic circumstances; in particular they point to the overwhelming importance of parental psychological well-being for children's well-being. Parental, especially maternal, psychological health affects the developing child directly, through the parent's capacity to provide care, emotional warmth and stimulation. Lack of parental care and a lack of emotional warmth, for example through parental mental illness, substance abuse or alcoholism are powerful risk factors for developmental and mental health problems, and have been found to serve as vulnerability factors for depression and as direct risk factors for conduct disorders and personality disturbance (Cleaver *et al.* 1999; Farrington and West 1981). A history of physical abuse in childhood increases the likelihood of lifetime psychopathology; this association appears stronger for women than men (MacMillan *et al.* 2001). In their community sample in Ontario, the authors found that those reporting a history of childhood physical abuse had significantly higher lifetime rates of anxiety disorders, alcohol abuse and anti-social behaviour and, for women in particular, major depression. As well as maltreatment and inter-parental violence, exposure to community violence can have internalising and externalising effects, putting children at risk for a range of emotional, cognitive, social and behavioural problems, depending on their age and stage of development (Margolin and Gordis 2000). At different stages, children face different developmental challenges that can be disrupted by abuse and violence.

The psychological health of parents can also have a less direct impact on the developing child, through the quality of the parents' relationship and their negotiation of the social and economic conditions in which family life is played out. The higher rates of marital and family discord that accompany parental mental illness negatively affect child development (e.g. Beardslee and Wheelock 1994; Rutter 1990). Social and economic pressures, and a lack of social support, place additional strains on the care-giving capacities of psychologically vulnerable parents and on family relationships. This means that parents with mental health problems face difficulties in caring for their children that stem from their illness, from social responses to their illness and from a generalised social exclusion. Unemployment, housing problems, poverty and the stigma attached to mental illness, increase the pressure on parents whose mental health is fragile. They often struggle financially and they are likely to live in social isolation.

The difficulties faced by children with a mentally ill parent are therefore very complex, depending on such factors as the nature and severity of the parental illness and associated psycho-social risk factors, including the resources of the wider family, as well as on the services provided for them (Göpfert *et al.* 2002; Hetherington *et al.* 2001; Reder *et al.* 2000; Rutter 1989; Weir and Douglas 1999). At the very least, these children are likely to experience disruption of their lives and anxieties about their own future mental health. In the most acute cases their own lives are at risk (Falkov 1996; Ramsay *et al.* 1998; Reder and Duncan 1999; Stroud 1997). The impact of parental mental illness on child health, welfare and development is well documented. Research studies have reported a range of possible effects of parental mental ill health on children, including the risk of emotional and physical harm, under-stimulation, developmental delay, neglect, isolation and subsequent disturbances in the child, both in the short term and longer term, into adolescence and adulthood. Children whose parents have a history of mental health problems are at greater risk of developing mental health problems themselves (Beardslee *et al.* 1996; Cummings and Davies 1994; Downey and Coyne 1990; Henry and Kumar 1999; Oates 1997; Reder *et al.* 2000; Rutter and Quinton 1984). Having two parents with psychiatric disorders or having one parent with co-morbid diagnosis increases these risks. In addition, these children may have to take on practical and emotional responsibilities for the care of their parents and siblings which can place emotional and social strains on normal developmental processes and which often go unnoticed by service providers (Dearden and Becker 2000; Frank 1995).

Recent epidemiological evidence confirms the significance of parent mental health, parental relationships and family functioning for children's well-being: in a recent survey of children's mental health problems in the UK, children with mental health problems were twice as likely to be part of discordant families, with 43 per cent of the conduct-disordered children in the survey coming from families with high levels of family discord (Meltzer *et al.* 2000). Parental separation and divorce, similarly, are risk factors for children, though it is likely that it is the conflict and hostility that often accompanies separation that are significant. There is also a higher prevalence of mental health problems in the children of 'reconstituted families', where children have experienced parental separation and remarriage (Audit Commission 1999; Meltzer *et al.* 2000). Lone motherhood too, was identified, in the same surveys, as a risk factor for mental health problems in childhood. However, whether it is the single status of mothers, or the interaction of associated social, educational and economic factors that poses a risk, as has been claimed elsewhere (McMunn *et al.* 2001), remains open to question.

There is substantial evidence that as with physical health problems, socio-economic disadvantage is strongly associated with higher rates of mental health problems, both in children and adults (Bradley and Corwyn 2002). Low family income, parental unemployment and low maternal educational levels have all been found to be associated with higher rates of mental health problems in children, particularly when they (typically) coexist. The disadvantages of poverty are more than material. Children of poor families are more frequently exposed to adverse life experiences, both in terms of life events and ongoing circumstances. At the same time, they and their families are often psychologically and socially vulnerable, lacking access to the non-material, as well as material, resources that would enable them to cope. These combined, and typically chronic, social and economic strains put these children at risk for a range of developmental problems, which in turn have educational, social and psychological repercussions.(Brooks-Gunn and Duncan 1997). Adversity, in the form of persisting, disadvantageous circumstances, can thus have long-term effects because of the ways in which it shuts off important opportunities and reinforces a chain reaction of risks throughout childhood and into adolescence. However, notwithstanding the clear evidence concerning the potential impact of risk factors, there is considerable variation in children's responses to adversity, and not all those who are exposed to psychosocial risk experiences succumb. In the next section we consider the concept of resilience and the factors which may protect children from the damaging effects of adversity.

Resilience

Children vary in their vulnerability to risk factors as a result of both genetic and environmental influences. There is abundant evidence that, in spite of apparently overwhelming circumstances such as those described above, some children are able to cope emotionally and go on to thrive in later years. Over the last two decades, more and more attention has been paid to identifying the features of these children's lives that enable them to be resilient in the face of adversity. Resilience refers to those processes, characteristics and mechanisms that enable the individual to resist the negative impact of psychosocial stress and to adapt positively to challenging circumstances and developmental threats. It has evolved as a construct with enormous potential, at a

number of levels, from individual interventions, to strategies and social policies to enhance and promote mental health across communities (Luthar and
Cicchetti 2000).

Studies have identified a range of personal and interpersonal factors which
are associated with increased resilience in high-risk children and young people.
Certain factors appear to protect children because they reduce the impact of
risk, while others promote resilience in the child through the development of
positive coping strategies. As with risk factors, they are located in the child, the
family and in the community. Resilience factors in the child include higher
intelligence, an internal locus of control, being female, having a problem-
solving approach and educational aspirations. According to Rutter (1985),
resilience probably involves several related elements in the child: a sense of self-
esteem and self-confidence; a belief in one's own self-efficacy and ability to deal
with change and adaptation; and, third, a repertoire of problem-solving
approaches. Interpersonal and family factors include secure attachment, at
least one good parent–child relationship, the presence of a supportive role
model and parental monitoring and supervision; community factors include
social support outside the family and educational opportunities and, materially, a higher standard of living and good housing.

However, the power of these factors to modify the effects of risk is not
straightforward or predictable. Research indicates that the mere presence of
resilience factors does not in itself determine outcomes. It depends upon the
nature of the risk factors involved, on the existence and interaction of other
protective factors, on the child's developmental stage and on the particular
'ecology' of family and community life, (see Luthar and Cicchetti 2000). To
some extent there needs to be a resilience–situation fit. In some contexts a
particular attribute is of less salience or protection than in another situation.
As with adults, an individual child has a better chance of coping if there is a
manageable balance of risks, stressful life circumstances and protective
factors; if the circumstances are extreme or persistent then the presence of
protective factors may not be enough to compensate, and even the most
resilient person will be overwhelmed. With this in mind, there is an emerging
consensus that, as well as identifying specific protective factors, it may ultimately be of more use to formulate risk and resilience as dynamic, relational
processes.

The study of resilience in development has challenged many negative
assumptions about children growing up under the threat of disadvantage
and adversity. It has been part of a shift away from deficit-focused models to
those that seek to understand and promote competence and, as such, has
much to offer mental health promotion. Some researchers even maintain
that resilience is common, rather than rare, and that it is made up of ordinary rather than extraordinary processes of adaptation. Masten (2001)
argues that this not only offers a more positive outlook on human development and adaptation but also gives a clear direction for policy and practice

aimed at enhancing the development of children at risk for mental health problems. However, notes of caution have been sounded about the conceptual and methodological pitfalls that surround the construct of resilience and the over-simplifying applications that have been associated with it (see Luthar *et al.* 2000). Nonetheless, there is general agreement that the area of resilience holds great promise. By investigating and understanding the processes that contribute to positive adaptation, in situations where we might typically expect maladaptation, researchers, practitioners and policy makers should be better placed, not only to devise ways of promoting more positive outcomes in vulnerable children and adolescents, and those at risk for problems and psychopathology, but also to develop broader strategies to enhance children's mental health universally.

Implications for intervention

From the preceding discussion of risk and resilience, it is possible to formulate some guiding principles to help in understanding the causation of mental health problems and in promoting better mental health. In order to develop strategies to reduce the impact of risk and to increase children's capacity to develop into emotionally and mentally competent adults, we need to understand the complex interaction of risk and resilience 'in context'.

First, the evidence concerning risk and resilience points to the necessity of seeing the child in social context. Children do not live in social isolation: from conception onwards they exist in reciprocal relation to others. These 'others' are most obviously identifiable at the 'micro' level of family, but the family itself is surrounded by, and interacts with, broader social contexts. Ecological approaches, as exemplified by the work of Bronfenbrenner (1979), seek to understand the child and its development, in relation to, and as a part of, a 'nest' of interdependent systems which operate at micro, meso and macro levels. These systems include: the inner family; the close social network of friends and relations; the wider networks of work, school and community with which some (or all) family members have direct contact; and the broadest system of social, political and economic institutions which have direct and indirect effects on the lives of individuals, as children, parents, spouses, workers, and on families and communities.

From the discussion in the preceding section it is clear that the mental health of children needs to be understood in relation to these systems. We saw that some of the most powerful risk factors for mental health and other problems, as well as key sources of resilience, lie in the social environments of children at micro, meso and macro levels. For many of these children the problems are compound and difficult to disentangle, the products of multiple, interacting factors. In early and middle childhood it is in the micro and meso contexts of family, home and school that troubled children are most likely to be troublesome; with the broadening world of adolescence, personal difficulties and anti-social behaviour extend beyond home and school to affect, and be influenced by, the wider community. This points, first, to the need for interventions which recognise and take account of the ecology of the child, and, more broadly of childhoods. At the heart of this perspective is the acknowledgement that childhood is not a universal experience, but one which is culturally and historically variable Second, using an ecological approach not only makes it more possible for us to identify and tackle a range of psycho-social and economic risk factors; it also helps to formulate the relationships between different presenting problems, both in the individual child and among cohorts. Third, there is a cost-effective value in ecological interventions which can, directly or indirectly, address several types of problem at once, for example by raising levels of supportive resources. Critically, if mental health, as part of general well-being, is to be promoted, it is vital that ecologies of resilience are nurtured.

The second principle concerns the importance of placing the problems of children and adolescents in a developmental context. Children are not static entities but dynamic, interacting and developing beings with changing developmental needs and capacities. The ways in which they respond to their social environment and how they experience and convey their distress depend upon their age and developmental stage. As we have seen, the impact of risk factors is determined both by the nature of the risk and the child's ability to deal with it. These vary according to the child's age and stage, thus risk and resilience take different forms during the course of childhood from infancy to adolescence. Crucially, some psychosocial experiences are most threatening to mental health if they occur at particular stages of development, with early childhood being a time of greatest vulnerability. In order to understand the potential impact of different factors on the child, we must take account of the timing of their occurrence and risk factors need to be mapped on to the appropriate developmental period. Though the consensus is 'the earlier the better', there is increasing agreement that a range of approaches should be in place for the longer-term of childhood; for those children who face the greatest adversity and disadvantage, multiple risk factors typically persist over time and through the major developmental transitions of childhood and adolescence. If we are to adopt a developmentally informed approach to the timing and process of interventions, whether oriented towards treatment, prevention or promotion, it is essential that epidemiological and clinical data are allied closely with developmental knowledge.

Combining these two principles – of understanding mental health in relation to both the social and developmental contexts of childhood – points towards the need for mental health promotion strategies at micro, meso and macro levels that seek to reduce risk factors and to foster resilience in developmentally appropriate ways. Strategic interventions through primary and community care and education, together with public health approaches, can be complementary. There are a number of strategies along these lines that are proving to be fruitful. Drawing on Rutter (1990) they are usefully summarised in *Bright Futures* as follows: reducing the risk by acting on the nature of the risk factor itself or altering the exposure to and involvement in the risk; reducing the likelihood of negative chain reactions arising from the risk; promoting self-esteem and self-efficacy through the availability of secure and supportive relationships, or success in achieving tasks; opening up new and positive opportunities and offer turning points, where a risk path may be re-routed (MHF, 1999: 10; for further discussion see Cicchetti and Toth 2000; Gladstone and Beardslee 2000; Rutter 1990, 1999; Tiet *et al.* 1998).

The family and school constitute the key social contexts throughout childhood and there is agreement that mental health promotion which focuses on these can, and should, operate at different levels. For example, given the vital association between pro-social behaviour and mental health, fostering social and emotional development is a significant key to improvement. The quality of social relationships in both family life and school life can be targeted at the micro-level of face-to-face interactions, from early infancy or before; at the systemic level of the family or school through interventions designed to address family, classroom or whole-school functioning; as part of a community-wide strategy endorsed by families and local health, welfare and education services and as government policy, through funded nationwide initiatives.

Family life, especially parenting and parent–child relationships, has been the object of a numerous local and national strategies in many countries, especially in the half-century since John Bowlby's 1951 WHO monograph raised awareness of the critical importance of secure attachment and parental sensitivity for emotional development. Research indicates that the resilience of children may be enhanced by secure and nurturing attachments to a small number of caregivers, and that this is more likely to happen if support is provided to parents and other caregivers, to enable them to build their confidence and skills in child care and their self-esteem (Child Psychotherapy Trust 1999). Sure Start in the UK is a recent government-funded, nationwide initiative, implemented at the level of local communities, which aims to increase parental awareness of children's needs and capacities, and to support them by providing skills training, family support and healthcare. In line with the 'earlier is better' consensus, interventions to improve parenting generally target parents with babies and pre-school children, though increasing attention is now also being paid to raising awareness and improving the parenting skills of prospective parents, both during pregnancy and pre-conceptually (MHF 1999). The Parent Adviser Service is part of a community child and family mental health service in Southwark, a south London borough with high rates of disadvantage (Day and Davis 1999). As part of its strategy to develop community-based mental health promotion and prevention, the service introduced a range of interventions to promote parent's abilities to care for the psychosocial development of their children, to enhance parent's self-esteem, and to prevent parental and child problems. The Parent Adviser Service provides home-based support for parents of pre-school children with psychosocial problems. This is carried out by health visitors specially trained in the skills of parent counselling, parenting and child behaviour management. The key ethos of the parent adviser model is the support and empowerment of parents to use their own resources effectively to manage their difficulties; the aim is to enable parents to build up their self-esteem, parental confidence and skills (Day and Davis 1999). At a more preventative level, this community child and family mental health service introduced a project in which health visitors conduct promotional interviews before and immediately after all new births, screen for families at risk of developing child mental health problems, and work intensively and immediately with those identified as being in need. A vital ingredient of primary care interventions such as these is thorough training and awareness-raising among staff, particularly in relation to healthy development, mental health and the importance of good-enough parenting.

While interventions with parents and children most typically target families with young children, research in the United States indicates that working with at-risk adolescents and their parents can have beneficial effects which are both ameliorative and protective, enhancing the young person's resilience. The innovative and influential research by William Beardslee and his colleagues, on preventative interventions for depression in children and young people, has focused particularly on families with parental affective disorder, a significant risk factor for depression in children. This work, over the last twenty years, has emphasised the importance of designing developmentally appropriate interventions, involving parents and children, which both promote resilient traits and modify the risk factors associated with parental affective illness. While the focus of Beardslee's work has been the development of adolescent self-understanding, family communication and functioning, he argues strongly that prevention of depression also requires addressing broader social adversity and therefore the adoption of public health models that seek to minimise social and economic risk factors (Beardslee and Gladstone 2001). A key feature of his research has been the indication that parental benefits from intervention are associated with significant positive change in their children. Providing opportunities for these young people to develop self-understanding and awareness, and for families to learn to talk about mental illness, appear to be important in the development of resilience (Beardslee 2000; Beardslee and Podorefsky 1988; Focht-Birketts and Beardslee 2000). In an extension of Beardslee's approach, in Sweden, the Netherlands and Australia, groups for children with mentally ill parents have expanded nationally, from local beginnings (Rimington et al. 1999; Skerfving 1999). In the UK, the Mental Health

Foundation has carried out a number of school-based projects from primary school to adolescence, which include peer support for children who show signs of vulnerability to mental health problems (MHF 2002). The common feature of this work with children is that the groups serve as a forum for meeting and supporting peers, learning to trust and talk with others about experiences and worries, building self-esteem and accessing information about mental illness.

School as a major feature in children's lives, has the potential to be a key setting for mental health promotion and for making help accessible to children who otherwise would not receive support. As well as formal teaching and learning, school plays an important part in socialising children as individuals and as members of a community. It is therefore ideally placed for a range of interventions to improve mental health and to foster emotional and psychological well-being (Durlak 1995). In her review of the influences of school on children's development, Sylva (1994) concludes that schools are central to the promotion of long-term outcomes. She suggests that many effects of schooling may be indirect, related to changes in motivation, self-concepts and beliefs about success. As we have seen, there are significant associations between educational achievement and emotional well-being. Children with learning difficulties, either because of low IQ or a specific learning disorder are at increased risk of mental health problems and those with mental health problems are much more likely to have special educational needs. More generally, there is evidence that children learn more effectively if they are happy in their work, believe in themselves, like their teachers and feel that school is supporting them. Equally, educational achievement can be an important ingredient in improved self-esteem (Weare 1999).

There are several direct and indirect ways in which mainstream schools at primary and secondary level can promote mental health and a range of projects in the USA, Europe, Australia and the Indian subcontinent demonstrate the effectiveness of school-based interventions for children of different ages. These studies point to the importance of supporting social and emotional as well as educational development, and of the particular value in addressing these kinds of difficulties among vulnerable pupils. Much of the work reflects an ecological perspective, attending to several levels of influence – whole-school, classroom, peer group and the individual – and some include parents and parenting (for examples see Barnes 1998; Cowling 1999; MHF 1999, 2001). In an early, influential project, the Yale New Haven Primary Prevention programme aimed to increase awareness in the school environment of a range of mental health issues, such that they became integral components of the school experience. Using an ecological perspective, the programme was based on the principle that cognitive and socio-emotional development are strongly interrelated, and a school environment, including its management, organisation, teachers and parents, can create the right climate for students to achieve academic success and mental health (Comer 1985). Tackling common mental health issues through the curriculum can play a useful part in raising awareness and de-stigmatising and 'normalising' mental health problems. This approach typically means educating teachers as well as their pupils, as for example the 'Knowing the Blues' Depression Awareness Project, developed in Monash, Eastern Australia, which is designed to involve pupils, parents and teachers and the consultative help of a community-based mental health service, in raising knowledge and awareness of depression. Targeting young adolescents in year groups, the project focuses on the vital importance of emotional awareness as a central factor in mental health and aims to equip young people with the knowledge and skills needed to address depressive symptoms, sooner rather than later (Lowndes 2001). In rural areas of Pakistan, Mubbashar *et al.* (1989 in Rahman *et al.* 2000) developed a school mental health programme which aimed to introduce mental health principles to improve the learning environment, to increase mental health awareness among children and teachers, and to train teachers and primary healthcare professionals to manage such mental health problems. Similarly, programmes undertaken in India have employed a range of approaches to improve the school environment through awareness-raising among teachers, parents and children (Kapur 1997, cited in Rahman *et al.* 2000).

At the whole-school level, there has been increasing interest in recent years in ways of improving the social and emotional life of the school as a community, by establishing a safe and positive school environment. This has been the focus of whole-school behaviour plans adopted in the UK over the last decade, in both primary and secondary schools. Whole-school approaches aimed at reducing bullying, such as those developed in the influential work of Olweus (1994) have been found not only to reduce the incidence of bullying, but also more generally to improve the social climate of the school, creating a warmer more positive social environment which sets firm limits on unacceptable behaviour. At the classroom level, interventions are aimed at improving the social environment of the classroom, reducing anti-social and disruptive behaviour and encouraging positive peer relationships. Working with children at a more micro-level, whether individually or in small groups, can enhance self-esteem, self-confidence and social relationships, to the benefit of the child and the social environment of the classroom or wider school (MHF 2001).

Conclusions

Adopting an ecological approach to promoting children's mental health means setting not only children, but also their environments, 'in context'. It is widely agreed that parents and other significant caregivers constitute the most vital element in children's development – and as such they provide the key to nurturing mental health. Parenting as a dynamic compound of emotion, attachment, skills and motivation, itself takes place in social, economic and individual biographical contexts. When these contexts are characterised by adversity, good-enough parenting is jeopardised. Strategies to improve parenting therefore need to recognise that parents, especially the most vulnerable, need support. If parenthood is reduced to merely a set of 'parenting skills', without recognising the complexity of the role and the often challenging conditions in which it is played out, then interventions are unlikely to have long-lasting effects. As well as programmes to tackle social inequalities and to minimise economic and social risk factors, it is clear from this discussion that enhancing the conditions of parenthood must involve wide-scale strategies to promote public awareness of the vital importance of parents and parenting in the development of children's emotional well-being and mental health. This also means raising awareness among children as future parents. Preparation and support for parenthood should be widespread and accessible, a standard, normative feature of support for development from child to adult. Wider acknowledgement that parenthood is not only a vital role but also, at times, a very difficult one, may make it easier for parents to ask for and receive help. Support which is responsive to parents, together with the involvement of professionals whom they can trust, can help to de-stigmatise help-seeking and enable early intervention (Baistow and Hetherington 1998; Phillips and Hugman 1999). Amplifying the debates about long working hours and parenthood, especially mother-hood, and encouraging or inducing employers to humanise working conditions to favour family *and* organisational life, rather than assuming that they are inevitably in opposition to one another, can help to raise awareness, as a basis for change.

Similarly, if we want schools, teachers, and health and social workers to recognise the intimate connections between cognitive, social and emotional development, and to use this understanding in their practice, then they have to be supported in doing so. The interventions in primary care and in schools that have been described above highlight the key role that awareness-raising plays in mental health promotion. It is clear that a range of professionals – teachers, health visitors, social workers, family support workers and general practitioners – need more knowledge and under-standing of mental health and illness if they are to work with children and parents in their 'natural contexts' to improve the emotional lives of children. But, in addition to training and awareness-raising about child development and mental health, and designing programmes and interventions to enhance resilience, practitioners need to be able to operate in contexts that make their implementation possible. Pressure of time and competing commitments, and the demands of short-term 'targets' and 'initiatives' – all common to the public sector in England – leave little time, energy or resources for slower, more thorough, collaborative work, which necessarily involves longer-term processes and outcomes (Baistow and Hetherington 2002). Of course, in a world of diminishing resources, there may be an argument for finding ways of enhancing the resilience of professionals to function in the face of adversity. However, there is little doubt that there need to be fundamental conceptual and practical shifts if children's mental health and development are to be seen as important community concerns, not only the responsibility of parents. Promotion of mental health and prevention of disturbance require early and long-term commitment at local and national levels if they are to have long-lasting effects.

As we have seen, children's mental health problems provide powerful reminders of the interrelatedness of human characteristics, which in health discourses and practice have so often become fragmented and separated. Reintegrating our thinking and actions with regard to mental health has implications for our understanding of the 'whole' person; but adopting a holistic approach also applies to the community – there is a critical social value in understanding the person in relation to others, for the sake of community as well as the individual. Further, placing the child or parent in context, at micro and macro levels, means more than taking a 'snapshot' of present conditions; it also means heeding the temporal, dynamic features of human existence. Individuals develop and evolve and so do communities. Thus, however much holism may be an attractive ethic, trying to practise it gives rise to the kinds of complications and uncertainties that 'policies' and 'programmes' rarely allow for. (Re)connecting our interests in mental health also means reviewing the segmented way in which we have organised our responses to ill health. Following the 'divide and rule' principle makes health and illness *manageable*; treatment, care, prevention and promotion have become useful concepts underpinning economic considerations and activities, and the new managerial mentality focused on budgets, targets and outcomes which has emerged in recent years. However, these increasingly precise and narrow definitions hardly create the right conditions for either thinking or working holistically. The promotion of children's mental health is not a separate activity but one that can and should permeate discourse and practice in treatment, care and prevention (Beardslee and Gladstone 2001). Equally, as children's mental health is integral to other aspects of their well-being, it may be of little use to 'promote' it separately from other aspects of their lives. The efforts that are most likely to succeed are those that seek to enhance children's life chances and that recognise the interdependent nature of the well-being of children, parents, families and communities.

Acknowledgement

The author would like to thank Vicki Cowling and the Monash School Welfare Coordinator Network, Eastern Health Child and Adolescent Mental Health Service and Monash School Focused Service, Victoria, Australia, for making available material from their 'Knowing the Blues' Adolescent Depression Awareness Project.

References

Audit Commission (1999) *Children in Mind*. London: Audit Commission.

Babinski, L.M., Hartshough, C.S. and Lambert, N.M. (1999) 'Childhood Conduct Problems, Hyperactivity-Impulsivity and Inattention as Predictors of Adult Criminal Activity', *Journal of Child Psychology and Psychiatry* 40: 347–55.

Baistow, K. (1995) 'From Sickly Survival to the Realisation of Potential: Child Health as a Social Project in Twentieth-Century England', *Children and Society* 9(1): 20–35.

Baistow, K. (2001) 'Behavioural Approaches and the Cultivation of Competence', in G.C. Bunn, A.D. Lovie and G.D. Richards (eds) *Psychology in Britain: Historical Essays and Personal Reflections*. Leicester: BPS Books.

Baistow, K. and Hetherington, R. (1998) 'Parents' Experiences of Child Welfare Interventions: An Anglo-French Comparison', *Children and Society* 22: 113–24.

Baistow, K. and Hetherington, R. (2003) 'Overcoming Obstacles to Inter-Agency Support: Learning from Europe', in M. Göpfert, J. Webster and M.V. Seeman (eds) *Parental Psychiatric Disorder: Distressed Parents and their Families*, 2nd edn. Cambridge: Cambridge University Press.

Barnes, J. (1998) 'Mental Health Promotion: A Developmental Perspective', *Psychology, Health and Medicine* 3(1): 55–69.

Beardslee, W. and Gladstone, T. (2001) 'Prevention of Childhood Depression: Recent Findings and Future Prospects', *Biological Psychiatry* 49(12):1101–10.

Beardslee, W. and Podorefsky, D. (1988) 'Resilient Adolescents whose Parents Have Serious Affective and Other Psychiatric Disorders: The Importance of Self-Understanding and Relationships', *American Journal of Psychiatry* 115: 63–9.

Beardslee, W.R. and Wheelock, I. (1994) 'Children of Parents with Affective Disorders: Empirical Findings and Clinical Implications,' in W.M. Reynolds and H.F. Johnston (eds) *Handbook of Depression in Children and Adolescents*. New York: Plenum Press.

Beardslee, W.R., Keller, M.B., Seifer, R. *et al.* (1996) 'Prediction of Adolescent Affective Disorder: Effects of Prior Parental Affective Disorders and Child Psychopathology', *Journal of the American Academy of Child and Adolescent Psychiatry* 35(3): 279–88.

Bowlby, J. (1951) *Maternal Care and Mental Health*, WHO Monograph Series No. 2. Geneva: WHO.

Bradley, R. and Corwyn, R. (2002) 'Socio-Economic Status and Child Development', *Annual Review of Psychology* 53: 371–99.

Brandenburg, N.A., Friedman, R.M. and Silver, S.E. (1990) 'The Epidemiology of Childhood Psychiatric Disorders: Prevalence Findings from Recent Studies', *Journal of the American Academy of Child and Adolescent Psychiatry* 29: 76–83.

Bronfenbrenner, U. (1979) *The Ecology of Human Development*. Cambridge, MA: Harvard University Press.

Brooks-Gunn, J. and Duncan, G. J. (1997) 'The Effects of Poverty on Children', *Future Child* 7(2): 55–71.

Child Psychotherapy Trust (1999) *Promoting Infant Mental Health*. London: Child Psychotherapy Trust.

Cicchetti, D. and Toth, S.L. (1992) 'The Role of Developmental Theory in the Prevention and Intervention', *Developmental Psychopathology* 4: 489–94.

Cicchetti, D. and Toth, S.L. (2000) 'Social Policy Implications for Research in Developmental Psychopathology', *Development and Psychopathology* 12: 551–5.

Cleaver, H., Unell, I. and Aldgate, J. (1999) *Children's Needs – Parenting Capacity. The Impact of Parental Mental Illness, Problem Drug and Alcohol Abuse and Domestic Violence on Children's Development*. London: The Stationery Office.

Comer, J.P. (1985) 'The Yale New Haven Primary Prevention Project: A Follow-Up Study', *Journal of the American Academy of Child and Adolescent Psychiatry* 24(2): 154–60.

Costello, E.J. and Angold, A. (2000) 'Developmental Psychopathology and Public Health: Past, Present and Future', *Development and Psychopathology* 12(4): 599–618.

Costello, E.J., Angold, A. and Keeler, G. (1999) 'Adolescent Outcomes of Childhood Disorders: The Consequences of Severity and Impairment', *Journal of the American Academy of Child and Adolescent Psychiatry* 38(2): 121–8.

Cowling, V. (ed.) (1999) *Children of Parents with Mental Illness*. Melbourne: Australian Council for Educational Research Ltd.

Crittenden, P. (1995) 'Attachment and Risk for Psychopathology: The Early Years', *Developmental and Behavioral Pediatrics* 16(3): 12–16.

Cummings, M. and Davies, P. (1994) 'Maternal Depression and Child Development', *Journal of Child Psychology and Psychiatry* 35(1): 73–112.

Dawson, G., Ashman, S. and Carver, L. (2000) 'The Role of Early Experience in Shaping Behavioral and Brain Development and its Implications for Social Policy', *Development and Psychopathology* 12(4): 695–713.

Day, C. and Davis, H. (1999) 'Community Child Mental Health Services: A Framework for the Development of Parenting Initiatives', *Clinical Child Psychology and Psychiatry* 4(4): 475–82.

Dearden, C. and Becker, S. (2000) *Growing up Caring: Vulnerability and Transition to Adulthood – Young Carers' Experiences*. Leicester: The National Youth Agency.

Department of Health (DoH) (1998) *Our Healthier Nation*. London: The Stationery Office.

Downey, G. and Coyne, J.C. (1990) 'Children of Depressed Parents: An Integrative Review', *Psychological Bulletin* 108: 50–76.

Durlak, J.A. (1995) *School-Based Prevention Programs for Children and Adolescents*. Thousand Oaks, CA: Sage.

Falkov, A. (1996) *A Study of Working Together, 'Part 8' Reports: Fatal Child Abuse and Parental Psychiatric Disorder*. London: Department of Health.

Farrington, D.P. (1996) *Understanding and Preventing Youth Crime*. Joseph Rowntree Foundation.

Farrington, D.P. and West, D.J. (1981) 'The Cambridge Study in Delinquent Development (UK)', in S. Mednick and A. Baert (eds) *Perspective Longitudinal Research: An Empirical Basis for the Primary Prevention of Psychological Disorders*. New York: Oxford University Press.

Farrington, D.P., Loeber, R. and Van Kammen, B. (1990) 'Long-Term Criminal Outcomes of Hyperactivity-Impulsivity-Attention Deficit and Conduct Disorder in Childhood', in L. Robins and M. Rutter (eds) *Straight and Devious Pathways from Childhood to Adulthood*. Cambridge University Press.

Focht-Birketts, L. and Beardslee, W. (2000) 'A Child's Experience of Parental Depression: Encouraging Relational Resilience in Families with Affective Illness', *Family Process* 39(4): 417–34.

Frank, J. (1995) *Couldn't Care More – A Study of Young Carers and Their Needs*. London: The Children's Society.

Gladstone, T. and Beardslee, W. (2000) 'The Prevention of Depression in At-Risk Adolescents: Current and Future Directions', *Journal of Cognitive Psychotherapy* 14(1): 9–23.

Göpfert, M., Webster, J. and Seeman, M.V. (eds) (2003) *Parental Psychiatric Disorder: Distressed Parents and their Families*, 2nd edn. Cambridge: Cambridge University Press.

Graham, P. (1985) 'Psychology and the Health of Children', *Journal of Child Psychology and Psychiatry* 26(3): 333–47.

Graham, P. and Orley, J. (1998) 'WHO and the Mental Health of Children', *World Health Forum* 19(3): 268–72.

Harrington, R., Fudge, H., Rutter, M., Pickles, A. and Hill, J. (1990) 'Adult Outcomes of Childhood and Adolescent Depression', *Archives of General Psychiatry* 47: 465–73.

Hayden, C. (1994) 'Primary Age Children Excluded from School', *Children and Society* 8: 257–73.

Henry, L.A. and Kumar, R.C. (1999) 'Risk Assessments of Infants Born to Parents with a Mental Health or a Learning Disability', in A. Weir and A. Douglas (eds) *Child Protection and Adult Mental Health: Conflict of Interest?* Oxford: Butterworth Heinemann.

Hetherington, R., Baistow, K., Katz, I., Mesie, J. and Trowell, J. (2001) *The Welfare of Children with Mentally Ill Parents: Learning from Inter-Country Comparisons*. Chichester: John Wiley.

Hofstra, M., Van der Ende, J. and Verhulst, F. (2000) 'Continuity and Change of Psychopathology from Childhood into Adulthood: A 14-Year Follow-Up Study', *Journal of the American Academy of Child and Adolescent Psychiatry* 39: 850–8.

Knapp, M., Scott, S. and Davies, J. (1999) 'The Cost of Anti-Social Behaviour in Younger Children', *Clinical Child Psychology and Psychiatry* 4(4): 457–73.

Kurtz, Z. (1996) *Treating Children Well*. London: Mental Health Foundation.

Lowndes, J. (2001) *Adolescent Awareness Project*. Maroondah, Australia: Maroondah Hospital and Monash Student Welfare Coordinating Network.

Luthar, S. and Cicchetti, D. (2000) 'The Construct of Resilience: Implications for Interventions and Social Policies', *Development and Psychopathology* 12(4): 857–85.

Luthar, S., Cicchetti, D. and Becker, B. (2000) 'The Construct of Resilience: a Critical Evaluation and Guidelines for Future Work', *Child Development* 7(3): 543–62.

Macdonald, W. and Bower, P. (2000) 'Child and Adolescent Mental Health and Primary Care: Current Status and Future Directions', *Current Opinion in Psychiatry* 13(4): 369–73.

MacMillan, H.L., Fleming, J.E., Streiner, D.L. *et al.* (2001) 'Childhood Abuse and Lifetime Psychopathology in a Community Sample', *American Journal of Psychiatry* 158(11): 1878–83.

McCann, J. (1996) 'Prevalence of Psychiatric Disorders in Young People in the Care System', *British Medical Journal* 313: 1529–30.

McGuire, J. and Earls, F. (1991) 'Prevention of Psychiatric Disorders in Early Childhood', *Journal of Child Psychology and Psychiatry and Allied Disciplines* 32(1): 129–53.

McMunn, A., Nazroo, J., Marmot, M., Boreham, R. and Goodman, R. (2001) 'Children's Emotional and Behavioural Well-Being and the Family Environment: Findings from the Health Survey for England', *Social Science and Medicine* 53(4): 423–40.

Margolin, G. and Gordis, E. (2000) 'The Effects of Family and Community Violence on Children', *Annual Review of Psychology* 52: 445–79.

Masten, A. (2001) 'Ordinary Magic: Resilience Processes in Development', *American Psychologist* 56(3): 227–38.

Meltzer, H., Gatward, R. and Ford, T. for the Office for National Statistics (2000) *The Mental Health of Children and Adolescents in Great Britain*. London: The Stationery Office.

Mental Health Foundation (1999) *Bright Futures: Promoting Children and Young People's Mental Health*. London: MHF.

Mental Health Foundation (2001) *Promoting Mental Health in Primary Schools*. London: MHF.

Mental Health Foundation (2002) Peer Support Website www.mentalhealth.org.uk/peer/

Meyers, R. (1992) *The Twelve who Survive*. London: Routledge.

Murray, C.J. and Lopez, A.D. (1997) 'Alternative Projections of Mortality and Disability by Cause 1990–2020: Global Burden of Disease Study', *The Lancet* 349: 1498–504.

Oates, M. (1997) 'Patients as Parents: The Risk to Children', *British Journal of Psychiatry* 170 (Suppl. 32): 22–7.

Offord, D., Szatmari, P. *et al.* (1987) 'Ontario Child Health Study: Six Month Prevalence of Disorder and Rates of Service Utilization', *Archives of General Psychiatry* 44: 832–6.

Olweus, D. (1994) 'Annotation: Bullying at School: Basic Facts and Effects of a School Based Intervention Program', *Journal of Child Psychology and Psychiatry* 35: 1171–90.

Parsons, C. (1996) 'Permanent Exclusions from School in England in the 1990s: Trends, Causes and Responses', *Children and Society* 10: 177–86.

Phillips, N. and Hugman, R. (1999) 'The User's Perspective: The Experience of Being a Parent with a Mental Health Problem', in A. Weir and A. Douglas (eds) *Child Protection and Adult Mental Health: Conflict of Interest?* Oxford: Butterworth Heinemann.

Rahman, A., Harrington, R., Mubbashar, M. and Gater, R. (2000) 'Annotation: Developing Child Mental Health Services in Developing Countries', *Journal of Child Psychology and Psychiatry* 41(5): 539–46.

Ramsay, R., Howard, M. and Kumar, C. (1998) 'Schizophrenia and the Safety of Infants: A Report on a UK Mother and Baby Service', *International Journal of Social Psychiatry* 44(2): 127–34.

Reder, P. and Duncan, S. (1999) *Lost Innocence: A Follow-Up Study of Fatal Child Abuse*. London: Routledge.

Reder, P., McClure, M. and Jolley, A. (eds) (2000) *Family Matters: Interfaces between Child and Adult Mental Health*. London: Routledge.

Rimington, H., Forer, D., Walsh, B. and Sawyer, S. (1999) 'Paying Attention to Self: A Peer Support Program for Young People with Parental Mental Health Issues', in V. Cowling (ed.) *Children of Parents with Mental Illness*. Melbourne: Australian Council for Educational Research Ltd.

Rutter, M. (1985) 'Resilience in the Face of Adversity: Protective Factors and Resistance to Psychiatric Disorder', *British Journal of Psychiatry* 147: 598–611.

Rutter, M. (1989) 'Psychiatric Disorder in Parents as a Risk Factor for Children', in D. Schaffer (ed.) *Prevention of Mental Disorder, Alcohol and Drug Use in Children and Adolescents*. Rockville, MD: Office for Substance Abuse, USDHHS.

Rutter, M. (1990) 'Psychosocial Resilience and Protective Mechanisms', in J. Rolf, A. Masten, D. Cicchetti, K. Neuchterstein and S. Wentraub (eds) *Risk and Protective Factors in the Development of Psychopathology*. New York: Cambridge University Press.

Rutter, M. (1999) 'Resilience Concepts and Findings: Implications for Family Therapy', *Journal of Family Therapy* 21(2): 119–44.

Rutter, M. and Quinton, D. (1984) 'Parental Psychiatric Disorder: Effects on Children', *Psychological Medicine* 14: 853–80.

Rutter, M. and Smith, D. (eds) (1995) *Psychosocial Disorders in Young People: Time, Trends and Their Causes*. Chichester: Wiley.

Rutter, M., Giller, H. and Hagell, A. (1998) *Antisocial Behaviour by Young People: A Major New Review of the Research*. Cambridge: Cambridge University Press.

Scott, S., Knapp, M., Hendersen, J. and Maughan, B. (2001) 'Financial Cost of Social Exclusion: Follow-Up Study of Anti-Social Children into Adulthood', *British Medical Journal* 323(7306): 191.

Skerfving, A. (1999) 'The Children's Project in Western Stockholm', *Social Work in Europe* 6(1): 22–5.

Stroud, J. (1997) 'Mental Disorder and the Homicide of Children: A Review', *Social Work and Social Sciences Review* 6(3): 149–62.

Sylva, K. (1994) 'School Influences on Children's Development', *Journal of Child Psychology and Psychiatry* 1: 135–70.

Target, M. and Fonagy, P. (1996) 'The Psychological Treatment of Children and Adolescent Psychiatric Disorders', in A. Roth and P. Fonagy (eds) *What Works With Whom: Implications and Limitations of the Research Literature*. New York: Guilford Press.

Tiet, Q., Bird, H., Davies, M., Hoven, C., Cohen, P., Jensen, P. and Goodman, S. (1998) 'Adverse Life Events and Resilience', *Journal of the American Academy of Child and Adolescent Psychiatry* 37(11): 1191–200.

United Nations (UN) (1989) Convention on Children's Rights. New York: UN.

Weare, K. (1999) *Promoting Mental, Emotional and Social Health: A Whole-School Approach*. London and New York: Routledge.

Weir, A. and Douglas, A. (eds) (1999) *Child Protection and Adult Mental Health: Conflict of Interest?* Oxford: Butterworth Heinemann.

World Health Organization (1977) *Child Mental Health and Psychosocial Development*, Technical Report Series No. 613. Geneva: WHO.

World Health Organization (2002) *Mental Health Global Action Programme*. Geneva: WHO.

Chapter 7

Zimbabweans in England

Building capacity for culturally competent health promotion

Martha Chinouya

This chapter explores how Zimbabweans in England make sense of health promotion within the context of their global community relations and their traditions in modern industrialised settings. The inadequacy of individualistic approaches to promotion of their sexual health has led them to attempt to construct programmes grounded in these community relations and traditions within a modern industrialised context. The urban populations in Western Europe and the United States are essentially multicultural. A test of a health promotion strategy in such countries is how far it supports the efforts of the diverse groups of which these countries are composed to contribute solutions which address the problems faced by members of marginalised communities. If the strategy is supportive, global community relations and traditions can be resources for health promotion. Much health promotion treats global community relations and traditions as best left behind on migration. This is discussed in relation to HIV and AIDS, which, among Zimbabweans in England and 'back home', is predominantly heterosexually contracted. This is not to silence the gayness of the condition among this population, as there are Zimbabweans who have contracted HIV through sex between men. The key point here is that HIV among Zimbabweans living in England and 'back home' is predominantly contracted through heterosexual encounters.

HIV infection is now recognised as a global health issue and, with migration, is increasingly affecting family members and whole communities in dispersed geographical locations. In England, HIV and AIDS are increasingly affecting black Africans in general, and Zimbabweans, in particular. Using the words 'black' and 'African' and 'Zimbabwean' is a way of capturing the diversities, differences and contradictions as well as similarities among this population. The cultural diversities, differences, contradictions and similarities emanate from complex intersections of their 'roots' (i.e. place of birth within a Zimbabwean setting), 'routes' (migratory pathways) as well as a cultural heritage that is linked with the African continent and Zimbabwe in particular. This cultural heritage often yields fragmented meanings regarding their 'Zimbabwean-ness'. Because of these complexities regarding notions of Zimbabwean-ness, the author of this chapter, known among her peers and family as Zimbabwean, writes from a standpoint that is influenced by her own ways of knowing, experiencing and interpreting this complex juxtaposition of 'modernity' and 'tradition'.

Black Africans in England experience health problems against a backdrop of negotiating responsibilities to kin and community spanning continents: those responsibilities, involving intergenerational and intra-generational economic, educational and emotional exchanges, are their central preoccupation. Their health status, even if compromised by serious threats, is a secondary consideration.

This chapter begins with a discussion of research showing how globally dispersed kinship relations and tradition can disrupt expected flows of education regarding sexual health to young people in England. It then shows that communities are finding ways of drawing on their traditions as a resource to help each other to address threats to their health. In so doing they are socially constructing their 'tradition' in a changing global environment.

After men who have sex with men, black Africans are the second largest social group in England affected by HIV and AIDS. With migration to industrialised countries, Africans affected by HIV are increasingly leaving behind relatives and kin in their areas of origin, in Sub-Saharan Africa, where the rates of HIV are the highest in the world. This creates a complex and intricate web of family members in dispersed space, some of whom are affected by HIV (Chinouya 2001a).

In an unpublished PhD thesis, Chinouya (2001a) shows that, because of migration, parents and some of their children are increasingly settling in global metropolises such as London in fragmented family groups. It is not unusual for some children to be 'left at home' with kin in Africa, when parent(s) and children migrate. Two key problems emerge. Adult migrants are expected to take on major financial responsibilities for kin left behind, including their own parents, siblings and children. Family members left behind may well include those who would traditionally be obligated to play essential roles in the socialisation of the children who have migrated. Both of these factors have implications for health promotion of migrant households. Financial responsibilities are pressing on adult migrants with regard to the requirement to ensure the flow of remittances, while the children who accompany them no longer have access to kin traditionally designated to assist them in 'growing up'.

Members of the extended family who have central roles in the socialisation of children, including education on sensitive topics involving the meanings and rules of sexual behaviour, rarely accompany a migrating unit of birth parents and children. For Zimbabweans, *vanatete* (paternal aunts), *vanambuya* (grandmothers) and *vanasekuru* (maternal uncles or grandfathers) are key people within their complex kinship web(s). *Vanatete, vanambuya* and *vanasekuru* are responsible for imparting notions of gender to their nieces, nephews and grandchildren, and are morally contracted to talk to children about sex and sexual health (African Issues Group 1999; Chinouya 2001a; Shire 1994). They, not the birth parents, are expected to take the lead in imbuing children and young people with the appropriate values, knowledge base and attitudes regarding 'masculinity' and 'femininity'. Sex is considered to be so highly charged morally, that discussion of these matters between children and their birth parents is considered to be unacceptable. It would be considered to be disrespectful for children to discuss sex with their parents. Also, if there were problems within a sexual relationship, it was *vanatete, vanasekuru* and *vanambuya* who were morally obliged to intervene in the hope of finding a solution.

Within their global family networks, *vanatete, vanambuya* and *vanasekuru* are often left behind caring for children whose parents have migrated, or Zimbabwean grandparents increasingly have to care for children whose parents have died from AIDS-related complications. They provide such care despite stretched financial resources. Children left behind in Zimbabwe, act as 'connecting financial points' for *vanatete, vanambuya* and *vanasekuru* and their adult children, the children's parents living in London. These normatively shaped reciprocities and obligations constitute intra- and intergenerational family commitments (Chinouya 2002a). They involve costs and benefits that often render engagement in sexual health promotion agendas in England, among some Zimbabweans, secondary to their pressing everyday imperatives. How parents and young people who identify themselves as Zimbabweans make sense of health promotion interventions within this context of globalisation, is therefore key to this chapter.

The chapter aims to describe the challenges faced by sexual health promoting agencies in delivering interventions to migrant Zimbabweans in England. The challenges are described within the context of the HIV epidemic and the synergy between migrant Zimbabweans, academics and health promoters working with this population in England. The focus on sexual health and HIV is a deliberate attempt to highlight the problematic nature of delivering interventions to a population for whom these interventions are not their most pressing need (Chinouya 2002a). Some innovative models of engaging Zimbabweans in the sexual health agenda are described in order to encourage more culturally competent ways of working with this population. The next section describes how 'tradition' may influence the framework within which newly arrived Zimbabwean immigrants make sense of sexual health promotion interventions in England.

'Tradition, the way we were before we arrived'

Writing about 'Zimbabwean traditional' ways of knowing is highly problematic as 'tradition' is constructed, socially, spatially and historically. Tradition is not static but is reinvented by each new generation as it takes over the cultural inheritance from those preceding it (Giddens 1999). With reference to black Zimbabwean migrants, who are the subject of this chapter, tradition refers to the ways cultural 'resources' carried by a generation of migrants at the end of the twentieth century, shaped how they made sense of sexual health promotion in England. These cultural resources are described within the context of their understanding of intra- and intergenerational kin responsibilities. This shapes some of their ways of knowing about who can speak to whom about sexual matters. The word 'tradition' is used to refer to a moral framework which springs from 'what it was like before' migrating to England. This moral framework, need not, however, be frozen in time and space. Under propitious circumstances, it can be a source for creative problem-solving.

To locate children's experiences within this debate, it is important to note that modern discourses of childhood and children used by teachers, social workers and health promoters, emphasise that children should be told about matters affecting their lives, including the presence of HIV in their immediate environment. The word 'affected' refers to children who are living with HIV or have a significant other living with the virus. These discourses are rooted in conceptualising children as persons who should be treated as autonomous beings. The discourses have been encapsulated in the United Nations Convention on the Rights of the Child and the Children Act 1989. Within such discourses, affected children have the right to know and express their views regarding how HIV affects their lives. Parents, in this context, have an obligation to tell children how HIV affects them. The transmission processes of HIV, including both transmission among sexual partners and from mother to child, renders telling affected children that HIV affects them most awkward. Doing so can lead to discussing the source of infection, and thereby involves talking to children about parental sexual behaviours and sexual health issues.

Traditionally, intergenerational discussion of sexual matters was part of the education and support provided by *vanatete*, *vanambuya* and *vanasekuru*. Tradition specifies specialised spaces for doing so, such as the *padare*, a space designed for talking about *zwechirume* (male preoccupations). This would include opportunities for exchanging information about ways of improving sexual prowess (Shire 1994). Shire noted that information discussed at a *padare* was not to be transformed into gossip and men who did so were expelled from the group or sent on errands. *Vanatete* and *vanambuya*, had the task of educating males excluded from the *padare*, regarding matters related to sex and sexuality.

Traditionally, women, too, had their spaces called *chiware* where they exchanged ideas of how to make beads and play games (in bed with their partners) using beads worn on their waistlines. Beads had symbolic, cosmetic and decorative effects adding beauty to a naked woman's body. Beads were also toys that enhanced a woman's sexual aura and were at times believed to act as contraceptives. However, in some male-dominated Zimbabwean cultures, beads were also a form of social control, especially of married women, to keep them from 'straying'. Men who could tell the colour of a woman's beads were implying that they had seen her undressed body.

Difficulties in talking to children about sexual matters have been reported among non-African populations in the UK (Social Exclusion Unit 1999). This is considered to be a problem which health promotion must address. The absence of *vanatete, vanasekuru* and *vanambuya* among some newly arrived migrants presents problems when British health promoters assume that it is the parents' role to tell children that HIV affects them. Within their globalised families, London-based parents are now called upon to be the *vanatete, vanasekuru* and *vanambuya* to their children. Professionals expect that parents will take on the role of sexual health educators, in particular, if HIV positive children and young people are to be able to make informed choices about their sexual lifestyle as they negotiate transitions into adulthood (Chinouya 2001a). Children too, encounter cultural difficulties related to respect for those who are older than they, in discussing with their parents how HIV affects them (African Issues Group 1999; Chinouya 2001a). Health professionals feel called upon to encourage parents to be open with their children about sexual matters that affect their well-being. They rarely have the cultural competence to engage in the complex negotiations with migrant parents which would enable them to disclose to their children that HIV affects them, while maintaining silence on how the virus is transmitted (Chinouya 2001a). Having described some of the cultural background, the next section describes how health promotion has addressed the needs of Africans who are increasingly affected by HIV in the UK.

The academic gaze and health promotion

As a discipline, African Studies in Britain emerged as an adjunct to the British Empire, with a bias towards colonial history, basically serving the interests of those travelling to Africa as missionaries or in government services (Fyfe 1999). It was in 1991 that the category 'black African' was added to the census. Before then, the experiences of Africans in the UK were relatively under-researched and under-theorised by scholars. According to the 1991 census, black Africans constituted 0.4 per cent of the total population, and experienced marginalisation through poor housing and high levels of unemployment or underemployment. Black Africans were also said to be the most educated ethnic minority group (McMunn *et al.* 1999).

The 1991 census showed that the position of black Africans, including Zimbabweans, was fraught with contradictions. Though highly educated, black Africans occupy employment positions that often do not reflect their levels of education or experience. Also, although 1991 census data showed that black

Africans are the most educated ethnic minority group, and epidemiological data show that this population is increasingly affected by HIV, limited capacity for research has been developed or used within this population in planning for health. The word 'capacity' refers to the skills among this population in health research, planning and defining the research agenda. Their educational qualities have not been harnessed or developed in planning for health.

Current capacity does not reflect the potential within this population in light of their educational achievement and cultural resources. These are severely underdeveloped and under-used due to funding regimes. There are very few black African researchers developing theory and conducting academically rigorous research with migrant African communities in England. Africans are employed as 'recruiters' or engaged from voluntary organisations to access groups of research subjects that mainstream academics or researchers are unable to access. Africans are not prominent in setting the research agenda or in indicating how issues of sexual health are rooted in ordinary life. Hence, the 'other' documents what it thinks the sexual health issues are. This is largely without reference to Africans' experiences of living in England.

Prior to the 1991 census, there is a dearth of literature pertaining to this population. Researchers have often excluded Africans in their samples or, if included in research, they are categorised as the 'black other'. Sexual health research among this population is often buried in the 'grey' literature, unsustained and often unpublished in peer-reviewed journals.

Health promotion initiatives targeting Africans involve short-term projects, wholly focusing on sexual activity, with condom distribution a key component, without commitment to culturally competent programs of sustained intervention (Chinouya 2001b). Condom distribution is often divorced from the social context within which people make sense of such interventions. Further, with the dispersal programme, there are increasing numbers of Africans, including Zimbabweans, settling outside London, in areas where sexual health for this population is not a priority. In a study intended to map the challenges faced by providers in England in addressing the health needs of this population, it emerged that professionals outside London lacked cultural competency in working with Africans (Chinouya 2001b). It also emerged that most sexual health promotion practice was not informed by research and there were concerns that some models of intervention were 'transplanted' uncritically, directly from use in the white gay community into the African community. This was done without evidence about the sexual health promotion needs of Africans. The appropriateness of these interventions is questionable.

The programme for the dispersal of asylum-seekers, has created challenges for providers outside London, who lack evidence of what the needs of this growing population are. From the 1990s to the present (2002), most research targeting this population in England has been centred in London. Towards the end of the twentieth century, some health authorities outside London were collecting evidence through needs assessment exercises. Again, until the late 1990s, research among this population often used convenient samples, namely, people who are already accessing HIV-related services, and was often conducted by people working in community-based agencies together with hospital staff. Most of the research conducted before the late 1990s was qualitative in nature with service *providers* engaged in talking about *their* perceptions regarding the health promotion needs of this population. It was in the mid-1990s that Zimbabweans were identified as a population increasingly affected by HIV and AIDS. In the late 1990s, there was a slow shift, in London, towards collaborative work between academics and African-led community-based organisations. None of these 'African-led' organisations was 'Zimbabwean-led'.

Responses from health promoters

The health promotion needs of Zimbabweans are many and are often unresearched. Health promotion targeting Africans living in London, and Zimbabweans in particular, has most often been divorced from mainstream health promotion research, resulting in limited use of evidence-based interventions. Most health promotion methods appear to be based on models of intervention that place emphasis on congregating service users in public events (Chinouya 2001b), highlighting condom and/or leaflet distribution (National AIDS Trust 2001).

From the early 1990s, health promotion has mostly focused on addressing the unresearched needs of people who were living with the virus and accessing services in various organisations. These organisations have been African-led, white-led voluntary sector groups or statutory agencies. The phrases 'white-led' or 'African-led' are used to show how the shape of the epidemic has influenced the development of organisations. White gay men, who were at the forefront of those known to be affected by HIV and AIDS were, typically, the founders of white organisations or charities, and their management committee members were predominantly white, while the reverse remains true of African organisations (Chinouya 2001b). However, the representativeness of Africans accessing services and those who do not is relatively unknown, therefore the needs of those already using services cannot be extrapolated with confidence to the needs of African populations in England.

To help address and contextualise the needs of Zimbabweans living in the UK, the African HIV Prevention Framework (National AIDS Trust 2001), informed by the mapping exercise (Chinouya 2001b), recommends greater use of traditionally rooted modes of intervention and community settings to address behavioural and attitudinal change among this population. The National AIDS Trust (2001) and Chinouya (2001b) recommend cultural competency, using innovative models of intervention. The next section of this chapter will show how tradition has been harnessed and used innovatively with Zimbabweans living both within and outside of London.

Using cultural competency in research and health promotion

The *Mayisha* Study, funded by Avert, a voluntary sector organisation, was the first study in England that aimed at exploring the sexual attitudes of migrant African communities in inner London (Chinouya *et al.* 2001). The word *Mayisha* was drawn from the Swahili language and loosely translates to 'lifestyle'. The study combined ethnographic techniques, with the researcher, the author of this chapter, going to places or social venues where sexual health interventions and research could be conducted (Chinouya *et al.* 1999).

A key recommendation emerging from the *Mayisha* ethnography was the importance of 'following the population' in their everyday settings, rather than in bringing together groups previously identified as being composed of people using HIV services. Informed by results from the *Mayisha* ethnography, various settings (including baby-showers, hen nights, clubs, restaurants, garages) were identified where subsequently, questionnaires were distributed, yielding a sample of 748 African respondents. Among the *Mayisha* respondents were Zimbabweans, Congolese, Kenyans, Ugandans and Zambians. Results from the study showed that a majority of Africans (including Zimbabweans) did not perceive themselves as at risk of HIV. Most believed that condom-use was the group norm, that they could persuade new partners to use condoms and that they intended to use condoms with their new partners. Despite these beliefs, less than half of the *Mayisha* respondents reported condom use in their most recent sexual intercourse, and the majority of those who had a new partner had not used a condom with that partner. The *Mayisha* Study showed that it was feasible to engage communities in sexual health research. However, the *Mayisha* study failed to utilise an opportunity for delivering interventions to a population that had been 'hard to reach'.

Informed by the strengths of the *Mayisha* model (i.e. the feasibility of engaging communities) as well as the weakness of the model (the inability to capture an opportunity and deliver interventions) a new model of working, the *Pachedu-Zenzele* action research model, was born (Chinouya 2001c, 2002a). The words *pachedu* and *zenzele* are drawn from the Shona and Ndebele languages, respectively, the two main languages spoken in Zimbabwe. The words loosely translate to 'as a community' and 'let's do it on our own', thus capturing the spirit of communal engagement in sexual health interventions and research. The words are based on traditional beliefs regarding the spirit of being a member of *pachedu*. Being in a *pachedu* traditionally suggested that, as members, people had a communal responsibility for upholding confidentiality in learning about sexual matters. The *Pachedu-Zenzele* peer-led model aimed to deliver interventions and collect evidence about the level of awareness regarding HIV health promotion services and sexual practices, and to evaluate whether Zimbabweans in Luton made use of the resources that were distributed to them by their peers. The *Pachedu-Zenzele* project followed recommendations that emerged from the *Pachedu-Zenzele* ethnography (Chinouya 2001c), with the researcher, the author of this chapter, occupying the difficult position of being an 'insider' because of her Zimbabwean-ness as well as an 'outsider' because she was a scholar and was not resident in Luton. Her position as an 'insider' enabled her to explore the everyday life of Zimbabweans in Luton, while at the same time allowing the 'strangeness' of the setting to confer guidance on the types of interventions that would sit well and not disturb the status quo of making sense of everyday life as a Zimbabwean in Luton.

The *Pachedu-Zenzele* ethnography showed that friends were very important in making sense of an illness as it unfolded. Friends constituted a lay referral network, and provided direction through the pathways to the department of genito-urinary medicine. It also emerged that the everyday life of Zimbabweans in this setting was often characterised by a sense of busy-ness with little attention paid to the sexual health interventions that were locally available.

Based on Zimbabweans' ways of knowing and experiencing their everyday life, it was recommended that a team of *Pachedu-Zenzele*-trained peers should collect evidence of their sexual health needs and priorities, and deliver sexual health promotion interventions in homes, workplaces and colleges. A total of 290 home-visits were made by the peers, collecting evidence and delivering interventions, as well as evaluating whether Zimbabweans were using the resources (including condoms) given to them. From this work, it emerged that sexual health interventions for this population could not be divorced from the socially excluded context within which Zimbabweans managed their everyday lives (Chinouya 2002a). It also emerged that Zimbabweans who were *Pachedu-Zenzele* respondents were a 'sandwiched' generation, with complex global intra- and intergenerational family commitments. The concepts of intra- and intergenerational family commitments are rooted in group solidarity and reciprocities (Chinouya 2001a). Because of Zimbabweans emphasis on group solidarity, in her unpublished doctoral thesis Chinouya suggested that it would be exciting to explore disclosure of HIV within the moral values of *ubuntu-hunhu*, which highlight the values involved in respecting one another and rules for maintaining and expressing respect among group members.

The words *ubuntu-hunhu* are again drawn from the two main languages (Ndebele and Shona) in Zimbabwe. Thus, the moral values underpinning *ubuntu-hunhu* are rooted in collective responsibilities, respect and compassion (Mbigi and Maree 1995; Tutu 1999). These moral values, grounded in communal solidarity, are integral to everyday life. The philosophical moral fabric related to *ubuntu-hunhu* is being investigated within the context of health promotion, including disclosure of HIV status, among Zimbabweans in Southend by the author of this chapter (Chinouya 2002b).

In Southend, researchers, mindful of *ubuntu-hunhu* moral philosophies, have designed an *ubuntu-hunhu* action research strategy, to collect evidence of sexual practices as well as to bridge the gap between academics, health promoters and those involved in theatre arts among Zimbabweans, while at the same time delivering interventions. This is in recognition of the fact that most Zimbabweans enjoy theatre arts but at the same time are in need of sexual health interventions. The *ubuntu-hunhu* interventions are delivered by peers, who have received an *ubuntu-hunhu* training programme that incorporates research, drama and delivering interventions to others. It is the group's intention to reconstruct the notion of *chiware* (discussed earlier in this chapter) as a non-gendered space for peer support regarding how to make sense of sexually transmitted infections.

Again, the concept of the *padare* discussed earlier in this chapter has also been revisited and reinvented in London as a non-gendered space. The author of this chapter is the researcher on the *Padare* Project, which was funded by Camden and Islington Health Authority in London. The aim of the *Padare* Project is to collect evidence of sexual practices and attitudes, and service utilisation, among a sample of Africans accessing services in the London boroughs of Camden and Islington. Evoking tradition, in the form of a *padare*, was critical for this sensitive project. As mentioned earlier, the *padare* was (is) a place where people could speak about sexual matters and discussions in such spaces are highly confidential. Capturing the spirit of discussing sexual matters in confidence is the ethos of the *Padare* Project.

Conclusion

This chapter has shown the challenges faced in addressing the sexual health needs of Zimbabweans in England. For this population, sexual health is neither the major nor the only concern. Ways of knowing – shaped by traditional culture – have been described, and how traditional culture has become a resource rather than a problem in addressing Zimbabweans sexual health needs. The cultural resources brought with them in their migration include a framework for making sense of intra- and intergenerational family commitments across global boundaries. The author has mapped the ways in which the various components of 'traditional culture' have been harnessed and made use of in sexual health research and interventions with Zimbabweans in England.

References

Chinouya, M. (2001a) 'To Tell or Not to Tell? HIV Disclosure Patterns Amongst African Families Affected by HIV and AIDS in London', unpublished PhD thesis, University of North London.

Chinouya, M. (2001b) *HIV Prevention in African Communities Living in England: A Study of the Challenges in Service Provision*. London: National AIDS Trust.

Chinouya, M. (2001c) 'Life in Luton 1: Mapping the Sexual Health Needs of Zimbabweans in Luton', unpublished. Bedfordshire Health Promotion Agency.

Chinouya, M. (2002a) 'Life in Luton 2: Combining Health Promotion and Research among Zimbabweans', unpublished, Bedfordshire Health Promotion Agency.

Chinouya, M. (2002b) 'Life in Southend 1: *Ubuntu-Hunhu* Solutions, Mapping the Social Care and Health Promotional Needs of Africans', unpublished, Southend on Sea Social Services.

Chinouya, M., Davidson, O. and Fenton, K. (2000) *The Mayisha Study: Sexual Attitudes and Lifestyles of Migrant Africans in Inner London*. Horsham: AVERT.

Chinouya, M., Fenton, K. and Davidson, O. (1999) *The Mayisha Study: The Social Mapping Report*. Horsham: AVERT.

Fyfe, C. (1999) 'The Emergence and Evolution of African Studies in the United Kingdom', in G.W. Martin and M.O. West (eds) *Out of One, Many Africas*. Urbana and Chicago: University of Illinois Press.

Giddens, A. (1999) 'Elements of the Theory of Structuration', in A. Elliot (ed.) *Contemporay Social Theory*. Oxford: Blackwell.

Mbigi, L. and Maree, J. (1995) *Ubuntu: The Spirit of African Transformation*. Rundburg: Knowledge Resources.

McMunn, A., Brookes, M. and Nazroo, J. (1999) *Feasibility Study of the Health Survey in Black African Populations Living in Britain, Stage One: The Demography of Africans in Britain*. London: Joint Surveys Unit, National Centre for Social Research and the Department of Epidemiology and Public Health, University College London.

National AIDS Trust (2001) *The HIV Prevention Framework*. London: National AIDS Trust.

Shire, C. (1994) 'Men Don't Go to the Moon: Language Space and Masculinities in Zimbabwe', in A. Cornwall and N. Lindisfarne (eds) *Dislocating Masculinity: Comparative Ethnographies*. London: Routledge.

Social Exclusion Unit (1999) *Teenage Pregnancy*. London: The Stationery Office.

Tutu, D. (1999) *No Future without Forgiveness*. London: Rider.

Chapter 8

Contested macroeconomic policy as health policy

The World Bank in Ukraine

Eileen O'Keefe

> Although Russian and Ukrainian distributions of income and wealth are much less equal than they were during the Soviet period, they do not appear to be excessively unequal when compared to non-welfare-state countries like the United States.
>
> (Gregory 1997: 29)

Globalisation is a set of distinct, interacting processes which push in different and contradictory directions. Its many elements include a global debt cancellation movement growing simultaneously with a movement to extend a free trade regime in goods and services (Held *et al.* 1999). Since globalisation is not a single, unified process, it cannot be said to be good or bad for health. What can be said is that some features of its operation are unfair and need reform at the very least. Globalisation involves an ever more closely connected world which is profoundly unequal and disproportionately shaped by the power of regional trading blocks centred in the United States (US), Europe and Japan (Hirst and Thompson 1996). Global movements, developments and projects have implications for the promotion of equity in health (O'Keefe 2000). The World Bank is a pivotal global actor using a macroeconomic knowledge base for making sense of and intervening in the well-being of nations. This chapter invites the reader to ponder the position of the World Bank in promoting or damaging health. Questions have been raised about its accountability.

The World Bank's central mission is devoted to macroeconomic policy to reduce poverty. Its loan facilities are intended to promote economic growth in developing countries and those making the transition from communism. A subsidiary objective attends to healthcare. The macroeconomic policy has greater impact than policy on healthcare on health status and its distribution in populations. On this defenders and critics of market models of development are in agreement. Nevertheless, the bank's macroeconomic policy attracts less attention from health analysts than do its policies on healthcare (O'Keefe 1995). The bank's explanatory account of economic development informs the exercise of its function and operates as a regulatory framework for any country on the receiving end of its intervention. Its liberal explanatory framework encourages the extension of market principles and the integration of countries into a global capitalist network. However, there is considerable debate regarding explanation in macroeconomics, especially the use of a liberal framework which gives little weight to inequality or relative poverty (Wade 2001). There is also insufficient data that might help analysts to choose among competing explanatory schemes. Wealthy countries have a disproportionate input into global actors such as the World Bank, shaping the belief system by which they operate.

Controversy about the knowledge base regarding economic development should lead to insistence that global actors remedy the accountability deficit. In the past, the World Health Organization (WHO) could have been relied on as a focus for attending to competing explanatory frameworks. However, a conceptual and policy consensus between the WHO and the World Bank has recently emerged which has important consequences. Less weight is accorded to disagreement about the impact of a liberal economic framework on health than is warranted. The World Bank may use a mistaken explanatory framework or it may implement policies poorly. Countries on the receiving end of bank support pay the price directly if this happens. For instance, the transition countries of central and eastern Europe and the former Soviet Union have been identified by World Bank researchers as 'a fascinating social laboratory for reform in healthcare financing since the early 1990s' (Preker *et al.* 2002). They have concluded that, reform, even in those countries with the highest initial incomes, such as the Czech Republic, has led to less equity. But it is not just those countries reliant on the World Bank for funding which may be damaged through the pervasive influence of the liberal economic framework. If this contested framework turns out to be flawed, powerful countries may not escape the side- effects of the wrong-headed conditions for growth imposed on others. In the context of globalising trends, wealthy parts of the world cannot insulate themselves from the consequences of poverty and inequality. Poverty and inequality in developing and transition countries present security risks to the wealthy nations. Globalisation is a project rather than just a happening. There is nothing 'natural' or automatic about the extension of international economic integration using free-market principles. The form that globalisation takes 'has been strongly shaped by those with the power to make and enforce the rules of the global economy' (Woods 2001: 389). Wealthy countries have overwhelming capacity to shape the dominant explanatory framework (Yergin and Stanislaw 1998). Their power also enables them to negotiate protective respite from the rules which they enforce on economically weaker countries. When the steel industry in a wealthy country, such as the US, needs protection or their agricultural sector needs modernisation, as in countries in the European Union (EU), they can negotiate longer time-scales than are expected of developing or transition countries. World Bank activity in Ukraine reflects these issues.

The World Bank has been intervening in Ukraine to promote its transition from a command socialist economy to a market economy. This enterprise has centred on facilitating privatisation. World Bank initiatives to incorporate Ukraine into the world trading system identify absolute poverty as an unacceptable side-effect of market-based economic development and regard it as worthy of alleviation. Relative poverty is not treated as a problem requiring alleviation. Priority has been accorded to the transition to a market economy over a transition grounded in equity and democracy.

Development was addressed internationally in the late 1970s, through the World Health Organization assembly, whose members include countries at all economic levels, and where scarcity, including absolute and relative poverty, were matters of concern, and questions of identifying and meeting basic needs for health and healthcare were pressing. Starting from the determinants of health, WHO located policy for health within a social and economic strategy operating at local, national and international levels. It treated health as a productive resource for, rather than just a consequence of, economic growth. It treated the pursuit of equity in health status between developing and developed countries and within countries as a central objective and called for a 'new economic order' to promote such an outcome. This was expressed in the *Alma-Ata Declaration* in 1977.

The *Alma-Ata Declaration* highlighted the social production of equity. It focused on determinants, including those operating at transnational level, constraining voluntary action for health.

This initiative was the result of developing countries acting as important stakeholders in making sense of the world and in setting policy. It set down a bench-mark for establishing democratic consensus in contrast to the construction of knowledge dominated by regional blocs, multilateral agencies and corporations exercising economic power, but accountable to a minority of the world (O'Keefe 2000).

WHO commitment to equity: from hard to soft targets in health status

Consistent with the *Alma-Ata Declaration*, the WHO took a firm stand on the need for a new world order to address the social determinants of inequity in health status. The WHO European Strategy in the mid-1980s made its first priority timed targets to reduce inequalities in health status among and within countries set in a broad public policy canvas, including prevention of environmental pollution and reduction of spending on arms (WHO Regional Office for Europe 1985). This target calls for reductions in inequalities in health status 'by at least 25%' (1985: 24). It pointed to the social production of inequalities in health status through institutional factors that are intrinsic to the operation of society. This encouraged examination of the impact of major actors such as governments and business on health status. It encouraged a conception of health promotion charged with scrutiny of policy and institutional action upstream. Such scrutiny might require changes in policy, to reduce differences in health status among groups. This position treats relative poverty as a problem for health policy.

WHO and the World Bank: movements towards partnership

During the 1970s and 1980s, the WHO and the World Bank were seen by health promotion advocates to be far apart on policy issues. The WHO was agnostic about the place of market principles, while the World Bank was an enthusiast. *Health 21*, the WHO strategy for the European region, signals continuity in its emphasis on the contemporary relevance of the *Alma-Ata Declaration*, treating poverty as the key risk factor (WHO 1998). It counts income-related health gradients across a given society as injustice and a threat to social cohesion. It acknowledges that 'increasing globalisation of markets may widen the gap between rich and poor'. We are told that 'trade and agricultural policies should ... be realigned to promote health', that health impact assessment should be central to accountability, that countries should co-operate to establish regulatory mechanisms to minimise the potentially harmful effects of foreign aid and trade policies on disadvantaged countries. However, there is no acknowledgement that nation-states might have to engage with the policies and actions of global actors in the public sphere, such as the World Bank, International Monetary Fund (IMF) and WTO, and global actors in the private sphere, such as transnational companies, to achieve this. And there is no suggestion that they might find their capacity as nation states, even acting in concert, insufficient to make their voices heard effectively in these global organisations. The WHO signals discontinuity by pulling back from the earlier policy of timed, quantified targets for reduction of inequalities in health status. And the WHO has chosen to work in close partnership with the World Bank. This constitutes a major shift in global alliance building.

During the 1970s and 1980s the World Bank stood shoulder to shoulder with the IMF in imposing free market-based economic, financial and welfare reform on countries in short-term crisis or needing long-term development support. The emergence of the World Bank as a key player in healthcare policy became evident following its *World Development Report* of 1993 and its position as the largest funder of healthcare projects (World Bank 1993a) . The WHO's robust framework lost a significant amount of credibility during a long period of heavily criticised management and its strong emphasis on equity was overshadowed. Under the leadership of Dr Gro Brundtlandt, from 1998 the WHO emphasised feasibility and backed the poverty-alleviating growth model in developing and transition countries promoted by the World Bank. The commitment to the reduction of absolute poverty came to the fore, with relative poverty consigned to the sidelines. In light of the willingness of powerful actors within the World Bank, such as the US, not to address relative poverty on their home turf, it would be surprising if the bank could get support to do so abroad. Within the liberal explanatory framework absolute poverty is viewed as unacceptable, and legitimately targeted by aid programmes and safety nets. Relative poverty is considered to be a normal and acceptable by-product of a dynamic market-based economic framework, which, all things considered, improves health world-wide. Hence, increases in inequality should be acceptable when seen through spectacles supplied by the World Bank. The WHO and the World Bank now work together exceptionally closely, bound together by the WHO's commitment to leveraged influence through partnership with powerful organisations (Lerer and Matzopoulos 2001). This is evidenced by the constant interchange of personnel and the convergence on explanatory framework and policy prescriptions. The most dramatic example is the WHO *World Health Report 2000*, edited by the World Bank's chief economist (Braveman *et al.* 2001; WHO 2000a). This follows *Health 21*, which directly appropriates World Bank discourse in indicating that 'disadvantaged groups' should 'have access to social welfare through the provision of "safety nets"'. The newly forged consensus may be precarious. It exists despite considerable debate within the World Bank – not least among researchers from countries in transition – which includes critical examination of the market paradigm. Do global actors, and specifically the World Bank, operate to promote health? We consider the case of Ukraine, where the World Bank has been active since soon after independence.

Ukraine

Ukraine is a country of 50 million people. It has considerable natural resources, including minerals and rich agricultural land. Strong in human capital, its population has been described by the World Bank as educated to the 'highest technical and scientific levels' (World Bank 2000). Formerly part of the then Soviet Union, it remains closely linked to Russia. With an energy- intensive economy, half of whose energy came from Russia at a fraction of its real cost, it has since independence built up a major energy debt. This has enabled Russia to acquire Ukrainian companies via debt swap. Independent since 1991, it became a member of the World Bank in 1992. It is not in the queue for EU membership and has therefore not been on the receiving end of the extensive foreign direct investment experienced by Hungary, Poland and the Czech Republic.

As part of the Soviet Union, it could have looked forward to benefiting from the *perestroika* plan for health and healthcare proposed in the late 1980s (Davies 1987). This included elements highlighting improvement in the management of healthcare but also on prevention and health promotion. Hence, healthcare was to be improved by:

- changing medical training in order to support effective management of patients in primary care, to reduce extremely high referrals to hospital and long hospital stays;
- training doctors to focus on quality of care, including respect for patients and not just quantity;
- evaluation of district physicians 'according to the levels of morbidity and mortality, absenteeism and disability in their areas, not numbers treated'.

The proposed capital investment programme was designed to support a preventative strategy targeting the needs of women and children. Health promotion was intended to be based on recognising threats to health, including high levels of smoking and alcohol consumption, increasing drug abuse, two-thirds of the population taking no exercise and one-third being overweight. Reduction on armament spending was identified as the key mechanism to allow 8 per cent of national income to be spent on health by the year 2000.

At independence, Ukraine's social indicators were below West European averages, but better than middle-income countries elsewhere. Its economy was so intertwined with that of Russia that chaos ensued with the split. Output dropped in both agriculture and industry. Agricultural prices were kept down while input costs sky-rockcted. With 44 per cent of its Gross Domestic Product (GDP) devoted to social protection in 1992, the Ukraine spend was not out of line with allocations in Western European social democracies, but was generous by US standards. The government attempted to maintain social spending but in fact rapidly cut central funding on pre-school education, hospitals, clinics.

Poverty

Along with much of the former Soviet Union, Ukraine experienced a descent into poverty in general and a descent into child poverty in particular (Carter 2000). It experienced a rise in income poverty, increase in wealth and income inequality, worsening education, large increases in unemployment and underemployment, and increased national and personal debt. This was accompanied by decreases in life expectancy and an increase in death rates. Cultural consequences included demoralisation of family life and a rise in gender inequalities. Evidence of increased reliance on institutions to care for children led to worry about the impact of poverty on the capacity of families to care. The European Children's Trust reported that 'for Central & Eastern Europe & FSU in the 1990s, the number of children in poverty increased dramatically, so that it is now higher than for the other vulnerable group, the elderly'. Using varying definitions of poverty, incidence ranges from 30 per cent to 63 per cent.

Since independence, there has been a dramatic fall in the birth rate. Health status has deteriorated with increases in the proportion of population not expected to survive to age 60. Between 1986 and 1999, the life expectancy gap between men and women increased from 8.1 to 10.9 years (WHO 2000b). During the period 1992–5 the mortality rate increased by 14.4 per cent in Ukraine, while dropping slightly in the European Union. The increase in Ukraine was attributed to blood diseases up 39 per cent, cancers 4.5 per cent, injury and poisoning 23.2 per cent, respiratory diseases 32.1 per cent (World Bank 2000). Premature death from diseases of the circulatory system and cancers are among the highest in the WHO's European Region (WHO 2000b). Infectious diseases, such as tuberculosis, have re-emerged with 10 per cent of new cases annually estimated to be multi-drug resistant (Dye *et al.* 2002). Such infectious diseases have found a congenial breeding ground. This is dramatic in the case of HIV.

HIV/AIDS

Ukraine's low HIV prevalence as of 1994 was succeeded by large increases resulting by 1998 in the highest incidence among the newly independent states of the former Soviet Union. The 28,000 persons registered as HIV positive in 1999 were thought to be the tip of an iceberg estimated at 250,000 unregistered cases. Heterosexual transmission was expected to penetrate the whole population. A number of NGOs took the lead on HIV, while the Ministry of Health had no overview of this activity. Health departments were unable to afford tests needed to ensure blood safety. With the health budget under stress, the public health system has been in decline. With little treatment available there was no incentive to test or to be registered. HIV has been identified as a human rights issue in Ukraine, as disclosure results in discrimination in employment and access to medical care as well as social ostracism generally. Agreed for 2001 was a peer education programme focused on 2.5 million students. The transition has been described as including conditions which promote disease (EC-US HIV Prevention and Awareness Programme for Ukraine 2000). The conditions identified include increases in poverty, school expulsions, homelessness, unemployment and intravenous drug use. Rapid cultural change involved a reduction in the median age of first sex from age 20 in 1996 to age 16 in 1999. This was accompanied by increases in prostitution and economic migration. The European Commission view is a stark comment on the health impact of the way the transition has been managed, to wit:

> the current social and economic crisis has fostered the conditions that facilitate the spread of HIV, while reducing the capacity of health services to respond effectively.
> (EC-US HIV/AIDS Prevention and Awareness Programme 2000: 5)

This view coincides with the United Nations Development Programme (UNDP) noting that Ukraine's global ranking on the human development index (HDI) had fallen from thirty-first to eightieth place between 1990 and 1996 (UNDP 1997). The HDI is a composite measure based on life expectancy at birth, adult literacy and school/college enrolment, and *per capita* income.

Gregory (1997: 29) noted that both national government and global actors had failed to set in place conditions which might have smoothed the way for positive economic change:

> the creation of a new social safety net system has been accorded a relatively low priority by both national and international organisations...a mistake because other reforms cannot be carried through if there is a general failure of support for reform.

The absence of a safety net system echoed in the human services sector the single-minded priority accorded to privatisation of economic enterprises encouraged by the World Bank:

> shrinking government resources have been diverted from health and education, causing a spontaneous 'privatisation' of these activities to the detriment of the poor.
>
> (Gregory 1997: 29)

Commentators sounding the alarm about the impact of poverty and inequality on health were typically NGOs, such as the European Children's Trust or UN bodies such as the UNDP, whose conception of transition was more broadly based than incorporation into a global market economy. The UNDP argued consistently that transition to an economy using market principles needed to be buttressed by at least two other transitions: to the rule of law and to the development of civil society. Institutional support for the development of democracy and pursuit of equity were deemed to be essential.

Does the World Bank promote health in a transition country?

It was asserted above that the bank has two distinct spheres of activity which have health impacts. One attends to macroeconomic policy. The other attends to healthcare. The former has greater impact than the latter on health status and its distribution in the population. The bank's *World Development Report* (*WDR*) of 1993 is the generally recognised landmark in which the bank staked its claim to pre-eminence in formulating policy for healthcare reform (World Bank 1993a). That document was presented as relevant to all countries, but especially to those that were developing or poor. Its proposals were for public funding to be focused on provision of an affordable package of effective public health measures and essential primary healthcare interventions. The bank devoted its *WDR* in 1996 to the countries in transition from communism (World Bank 1996). It gave pride of place to market-based reform. Its prescription there was simple and clear: liberalisation and opening of these countries into the global trading system. This would yield benefits, including health benefits. Furthermore, this should take place rapidly. The World Bank's *World Development Report* for 1995 had set the scene, noting that 'despite the rich stock of human capital ... transition to the market has started with a collapse in production that has resulted in high unemployment' (World Bank 1995: 123). It noted as well a surge of corruption, organised crime and drug trafficking. Despite this, the policy it proposed was 'mass privatisation, falling trade protection, and a more workable financial system' (1995: 123). Treating globalisation as an economic process, rather than a complex and contradictory set of movements, the bank went on to argue that 'trade is the primary vehicle for realising the benefits of globalisation' (World Bank 2001b). Governments are urged to take steps to help workers displaced by this process to 'adjust'. This is justified because 'many workers will [wrongly] blame foreign trade for job losses and wage cuts' (World Bank 1995: 123). The *World Development Reports*, devoted to macroeconomics, shape the bank's lending strategies as well as providing kite-marking for foreign direct investment.

The World Bank has been active in Ukraine since 1992. Ukraine has been on the receiving end of assistance from the bank consistent with the macroeconomic framework approach summarised in the *World Development Report* of 1996. The bank's input has been two-pronged: reform of economic activity and reform of public sector provision. Public sector reform has always been the poor sister to the focus on macroeconomic reform. The bank's 1993 social protection strategy called for cuts to public spending, targeting vulnerable groups and improvements to the efficiency of the social spend (World Bank 1993b). Its starting point was concern regarding 'high spending on education and health inherited from the former Soviet Union' (1993b: 1). The principle of universal entitlement in contrast with targeted safety nets was considered to be unacceptable.

The bank carried out an analysis of its activities in Ukraine between the years 1992 and 1998 (World Bank 2000). The primacy accorded to market-based economic reform by the World Bank is evident in its funding priorities. Commenting on its cumulative funding as at January 1999 amounting to US$2.8 billion the bank asserts that 'The bank placed a high priority on privatisation' (World Bank 2000: 17).

It concluded that its intervention during this period was 'only partially effective'. Monetary stabilisation was achieved and hyperinflation, which was rampant between 1993 and 1994, was controlled. And 'good progress' was made with respect to privatisation: 47,000 small firms and 9000 medium to large-scale firms were privatised. To the bank's disappointment, few state-owned enterprises, less than 200, took this route. Good progress was also claimed with respect to trade and price liberalisation and strengthening of the central bank. Despite agricultural production falling to less than half and still decreasing and exports down, it judged agriculture to have achieved 'partial progress'. The list of areas in which 'little progress' was achieved is long. It includes:

- reforming the electricity industry and heavy industry;
- making the legal system transparent;
- reforming the social safety net system (starting from overly generous pensions and low retirement age, and benefits accounting for 25 per cent of GDP, at independence);
- reforming health and education.

The bank found that since independence the economic circumstances of the population were dire. It found wages down 35 per cent since 1990 and income *per capita* down by more than 40 per cent (1989–97). This was despite support based on what the bank took to be the correct analysis and correct identification of key issues. Deterioration was attributed to barriers to adopting the bank's analysis. The barriers cited included the following, all of which are internal to Ukraine itself:

- lack of political commitment to reform;
- lack of public consensus on reform: 'public cynicism about the transition reform agenda is high' (World Bank 2000: 24);
- absence of a business environment necessary for a market economy;
- self-contradictory commercial law and lack of enforcement;
- more senior management time devoted to licensing, inspection, rules than elsewhere: 'onerous regulatory environment ... interventionist public administration ... akin to the Soviet system' (World Bank 2000: 1);
- corruption;
- unofficial economy accounting for 46 per cent of the economy, the highest in the former Soviet Union;
- vested interests.

Despite the partial successes noted, Ukraine experienced a downward spiral. The bank summarised development outcomes as follows:

> living standards for most of the population have declined dramatically and poverty has increased dramatically since independence. The state benefit and welfare system has not been able to cope with this rise in poverty nor to ameliorate the negative impact of transition.
>
> (World Bank 2000: 23)

The conclusions from the bank's auto-critique were that it had the right ideas but did not manage to put them into practice effectively: 'the bank has often over-estimated implementation capacity' (2000: 23). It had not developed 'an operationally coherent strategy' (2000: 23). For a start, it settled for having its initiatives carried out in a wholly top-down fashion under emergency powers of the Presidency. And this against the background of grudging agreement of central ministries to deliver on conditions required by the loans. The bank had not managed to convince either government officials or other stakeholders of the rationale for the changes required. It did not try, for instance, to establish or nurture working groups, or to make contact with regional and sub-regional stakeholders. The bank concluded that this top-down approach should be replaced by ensuring that it worked in future at *Oblast* and local levels, as well as with central government. The bank depicts itself as a learning organisation:

'Today the Bank has a more sophisticated understanding of governance issues in Ukraine ...' (2000: 23). It indicates that in future it needs to include a 'fuller diversity of political and public administrative groups ...' (2000: 23) in its initiatives. No rethinking has been deemed necessary regarding either the liberal economic framework advanced or the health sector reform agenda. The key issue remains to 'reduce the role of administration in the economy' (2000: 23). The bank stands by its view that Ukraine still needs targeted safety nets softened by a 'more equitable support system for the poorest groups' (2000: 23). Poverty alleviation is acceptable but not a policy of broad or universal entitlement to publicly funded services. Its auto-critique does not engage with arguments regarding the impact of relative inequality on the distribution of health status in the population. On this showing, it would have little interest in the application to transition countries of insights regarding the relationship between relative poverty and inequalities in health status developed in Western Europe which researchers are engaged in exploring (Marmot and Bobat 2000).

A chastened World Bank notes that some of the proposals for development it previously advocated called for a strategy which was too much of a strait-jacket. The call for reduced welfare spending, more efficient welfare spending and severe targeted use of safety nets might backfire. For instance, overly severe targeting might lead those not eligible, to act to maintain their living standards, and in so doing take steps which reduce overall welfare, increase out-of-pocket costs or threaten exit. This point had been made repeatedly by NGOs, including the European Children's Trust, which had collected evidence that the position of low-paid workers, such as teachers, no longer eligible for state benefits, was not significantly better than those deemed to be poor enough for access to safety nets. The bank concluded that staunch commitment to ideologically driven solutions was inappropriate. On the basis of its experience of working in Ukraine, the bank offered what it saw as a less ideologically driven alternative for the future.

The more pragmatic solutions were to include the following ingredients:

* full participation of those being helped;
* ownership of solution by those most affected (World Bank 2001b).

None of this questions the original analysis or identification of key issues.

Following the auto-critique the bank carried out a study of poverty and social safety nets in Ukraine (World Bank 2001a). In light of the extent of the informal economy, its household survey examined expenditure, which was 37 per cent above income. Defining the poverty line as 75 per cent of median expenditures and extreme poverty as 60 per cent, it found that '26.7% of Ukrainian households were poor and 13.5% were very poor'. Factors protective against poverty for an individual were identified as a high level of education, preferable employment status, living in a small family with low dependency ratios and living in a big city. There are oddities in this study. Researchers note that 'refusals' to participate in the survey were high in big cities (42 per cent in Kiev) and low in rural areas (2.2 per cent in Zakarpatya) and that response rates were lower in the wealthy areas. Most importantly, the exercise raises a serious question regarding the extent to which it meets conditions the bank undertook when promising a less ideologically driven alternative. Bank researchers note that the 1999 law 'On Subsistence Minimum' established a minimum consumption basket for each age group (World Bank 2001a). The bank study group concluded that, since this cost more than the median expenditure of the population, the 'minimum consumption basket is not a practical alternative for this study' (2001a: 12). It went on to say that while this may 'reflect standards that Ukrainians would like to reach, it does not identify the poorest members of the community for whom assistance is needed' (2001a: 13). How does this relate to promises of 'full participation of those being helped' and 'ownership of solution by those most affected'? The study singled out a peculiarity of the Ukrainian social support system, namely the large proportion of the population eligible for military pensions. However, there was no discussion of what the meaning of this is within the culture, or what the consequences might be if this tranche of support were reduced as proposed. A new Programmatic Adjustment Loan followed swiftly for the period 2001–3. This holds no surprises and is wholly consistent with the recipes of the past. It is designed to strengthen financial discipline, put into place a regulatory framework for sustainable economic growth and to attract foreign direct investment. Key to this is the transfer of state assets 'to private owners as a corner-stone of the market economy' and measures to 'change the perception of the state as a benefactor'. To achieve the latter, pensions need to be carefully targeted. The bank's stated aim of extending social services to all, is to be achieved by the introduction of a carefully means- tested programme. The key mechanism for 'deep structural reforms' in health and education was seen to require the 'mobilisation of private financing ...'.

Ukraine in the world market-place: the downside of globalisation

Ukraine exemplifies many aspects of health as a global issue where events in one country impinge on the health of others. The best-known example is the case of Chernobyl in 1986, with the catastrophic explosion of its nuclear power plant. But macroeconomic events can present global threats to health as well. The poverty and social disruption following the fall of the former Soviet Union has resulted in the incorporation of Ukraine into world trade in many ways. This is not confined to the forms of trade welcomed by market enthusiasts. For instance, Ukraine has joined the world market in relation to the sex industry. This international trade includes the coerced trafficking of sex workers to the West, including to London (Kelly 2000).

The demise of major parts of the economy has reinforced the importance of Ukraine in the arms trade. It is now the seventh-largest supplier of major conventional weapons in the world (Stockholm International Peace Research Institute 2002). It has become active in the international illegal arms trafficking network as well. It is a key source, along with Bulgaria and Moldova, for the sale of arms and planes to Africa. This has included deals with Liberia, involving diamond swaps, which fuelled the civil war in Sierra Leone, as well as supplies to Angola, with UK companies prominent in brokerage (Bowcroft and Norton-Taylor 2000). It is ironic that the arms industry and the military actions which it provokes had been identified in *perestroika* initiatives and in analyses of obstacles to healthy public policy by the World Health Organization. The single-minded focus of global actors such as the World Bank, on a contestable macroeconomic policy, makes it easier for Ukrainians to make unhealthy choices. These aspects of market activity do not merit policy analysis in the World Bank auto-critique, motivated as it is by a narrow conception of development and globalisation. But they are not surprising to social scientists, who have repeatedly called attention to the complexity of globalisation and the downside of globalisation dominated by a minority of wealthy trading blocs. They have pointed to avenues opened through globalisation to desperate people who have lost out in these processes (Castells 1993). Rogers (2000) argues in his analysis of global security, that the 'gap between rich and poor is grotesquely excessive, is getting worse, and, as well as a threat to security, is an affront to justice'. He takes this gap to be promoted by the active structuring of the world trade framework to confer economic advantage on powerful wealthy countries which 'handicap' poorer countries. He argues that poorer countries will not be able to kick-start development in the absence of a 'radical programme of debt cancellation' or controls over short-term speculation. Researchers from the World Bank and the WHO, working together, refer to 'constraints' to health development all of which are internal to the countries concerned: low-level constraints include educational level of mothers, physical distance to facilities, user fees, lack of accountability to communities

(Jha *et al.* 2002). High-level constraints include: corruption, poor rule of law, armed conflict. Again these constraints are deemed to be internal to individual countries. There is no mention here of debt or protectionist trade action by wealthy countries in the EU, or by the USA, as constraints. This is an odd omission since debt has been singled out as a major constraint on prospects for sustainable economic development in Ukraine: a 'vicious circle of indebtedness' requiring debt service obligations has led to damagingly high reductions in spending on social and economic programmes and to 'excessive' exposure to volatility in financial markets (UNDP 1999b). External debt at the end of 1999 was more than US$12.8 billion.

The World Bank as a learning organisation?

Macroeconomic policy is widely accepted as impacting on health. This applies to those championing and those questioning the strategy of rapid incorporation of poor and transition countries into a free market in goods and services. Dispute is rife over the effects of economic policy on health. Among parties to this debate, the World Bank comes down strongly on the side of a liberal explanatory and policy framework. World Bank researchers studying eighty countries over a forty-year period, concluded that capitalism benefits poor people and does not increase inequalities in those countries which participate in the global economy (Dollar and Kraay 2000). In addition, they marshal evidence suggesting that public spending does not benefit poor people. At the heart of the World Bank, controversy regarding this explanatory framework has been rife. The author of the *World Development Report* devoted to attacking poverty (World Bank 2001b) is reported to have resigned from the bank because 'his emphasis on income redistribution brought him into conflict with other economists at the bank, who argued that market liberalisation was the most effective weapon in combating poverty' (Beattie 2000: 13). Easterly (2001), another bank insider, examined fifty years of bank theory, policy and practice with respect to developing countries and concluded that much of its activity had used overly simplistic market models and prescriptions. He found the World Bank to be 'lacking transparency, accountability and legitimacy ...'. Joseph Stiglitz, chief economist of the World Bank until early 2000 and recipient of the 2001 Nobel Prize in Economics, questioned the bank's enthusiasm for liberalised financial markets and aversion to active government involvement in the economy. He is reported to have left the bank in order to encourage wider debate about development strategies as well as the lack of power of poor countries within the decision-making apparatus (Patomäki 2001). One might have hoped that World Bank analysts were beginning to learn from critical colleagues that some of their key policy positions were questionable. For instance, researchers from the IMF investigated Eastern Europe and the former Soviet Union making the shift from central planning to market economies (Keane and Prasad 2001). They found that the typical pattern was that income inequality increased substantially during the first decade, that there was poor growth performance and that current GDP remained far below pre-transition levels. In the case of Russia, standard measures of income inequality had increased by 75 per cent and GDP stood at less than two-thirds of the 1991 level. Ukraine presented an even starker picture with more than a doubling of income inequality during transition and an average reduction in GDP per annum of 11 per cent. Poland was the exception. It was the only transition country with substantial economic growth: real GDP was 28 per cent higher in 1999 than 1989. While it experienced a marked increase in labour earnings inequality, there was only modest increase in overall income inequality. This was attributed to a major difference: a 'sharp increase in government cash transfers to individuals. In the first four years, transfers rose from 10% of GDP to 20%' (Keane and Prasad 2001: 53)

Outsiders are even more emphatic about the shortcomings of the bank. It is accused of being dominated by 'a technocratic elite of believers in the orthodoxy, backed by a few Western governments' (Patomäki 2001). The governance arrangements applying to global actors, such as the World Bank, do not take account of the range of explanatory and policy disagreement inside and outside the bank. Despite disagreement, the greatest weight is given to an explanatory framework that heralds a free trade growth model as the way to encourage health-promoting economic development. Wealthy countries have themselves become alarmed by recent economic and financial catastrophes in Mexico, South East Asia, Russia, Brazil and Argentina. This has led to G-7-led moves to redesign institutions managing global capital flows. Once again, these initiatives in cooperation with the World Bank and the IMF have found no space for representation of the economically weaker countries (Griffiths-Jones 2000).

The World Health Organization emphasises the interdependence of the world and the necessity for solidarity, and asserts that health should be treated as a human right. Its presupposition is that health interests are so interdependent globally that this makes sense from the self-interested point of view of wealthier countries. If the World Bank uses an inappropriate macroeconomic framework, it is not the wealthy who will be on the front line in paying the price. In fact, the outcome may be a lose-lose situation. Voices are raised indicating that the poverty and inequality facing developing and transition countries *is* a serious issue of security facing the wealthy countries. The downside of liberal globalisation includes increasing cross-border movements of refugees, terrorism, crime and disease. World Bank confidence in its knowledge base has ill prepared the wealthy countries for the whirlwind that they will reap. Disagreements on explanation regarding economic development indicate the need for decision-making mechanisms that redress the current accountability deficit which prevails at the heart of the bank. Redressing the accountability deficit would enable countries such as Ukraine to promote the health of their citizens instead of being objects of policy.

References

Beattie, A. (2000) 'Author of World Bank Report Resigns', *Financial Times* 15 June: 13.

Bowcroft, O. and Norton-Taylor, R. (2000) 'Africa's Merchant of Death', *The Guardian* 23 Dec.: 1.

Bravemen, P., Starfield, B. and Geiger, H.J. (2001) '*World Health Report 2000*: How It Removes Equity from the Agenda for Public Health Monitoring and Policy', *British Medical Journal* 323: 678–81.

Carter, R. (2000) *The Silent Crisis: The Impact of Poverty on Children in Eastern Europe and the Former Soviet Union*. London: The European Children's Trust.

Castells, M. (1993) 'The Informational Economy and the New International Division of Labour', in M. Carnoy, M. Castells, S. Cohen and F.H. Cardoso (eds) *The New Economy in the Informational Age*. Basingstoke: Macmillan.

Davies, P. (1987) 'Soviet Healthcare: Dawn of a New Age?', *Health Service Journal* 19 November: 1350–3.

Dollar, D. and Kraay, A. (2000) *Growth is Good for the Poor*. www. worldbank. org/research/growth/absddolakray.htm

Dye, C., Williams, B., Espinal, M. and Raviglione, M. (2002) 'Erasing the World's Slow Stain: Strategies to Beat Multi-Drug Resistant Tuberculosis', *Science* 295: 2042–6.

Easterly, W. (2001) *The Elusive Quest for Growth: Economists' Adventures and Misadventures in the Tropics*. Boston, MA: MIT Press.

EC-US HIV/AIDS Prevention and Awareness Programme for Ukraine (2000) *The Oblast Youth Prevention Project*. London: European Commission.

Gregory, P. (1997) *Russia and Ukraine*. New York: UNDP.

Griffith-Jones, S. (2000) 'Proposals for a Better Financial Architecture', *World Economics* 1(2): 111–33.

Held, D., McGrew, A., Goldblatt, D. and Perraton, J. (1999) *Global Transformations*. Cambridge: Polity Press.

Hirst, P. and Thompson, G. (1996) *Globalization in Question*. Cambridge: Polity Press.

Jha, P., Mills, A., Hanson, K. *et al.*. (2002) 'Improving the Health of the Global Poor', *Science* 295: 2036–9.

Keane, M. and Prasad, E. (2001) 'Poland: Inequality, Transfers and Growth in Transition', *Finance & Development* March: 50–3.

Kelly, L. (2000) *Stopping Traffic: Exploring the Extent of and Responses to Trafficking in London*. London: Home Office.

Lerer, L. and Matzopoulos, R. (2001) 'The Worst of Both Worlds: The Management Reform of the World Health Organization', *International Journal of Health Services* 31(2): 415–38.

Marmot, M. and Bobat, M. (2000) International Comparators and Poverty and Health in Europe', *British Medical Journal* 321: 1124–8.

O'Keefe, E. (1991) 'The World Health Organization European Strategy, Racism and the Alma-Ata Declaration', *Critical Public Health* 1: 36–41.

O'Keefe, E (1995) 'The World Bank, Health Policy and Equity', *Critical Public Health* 6(3): 28–35.

O'Keefe, E. (2000) 'Equity, Democracy and Globalization', *Critical Public Health* 10(2): 167–77.

O'Keefe, E. and Scott-Samuel, A. (in press) 'Human Rights and Wrongs: Can Health Impact Assessment Help?', *Journal of Law, Medicine & Ethics.*

Patomäki, H. (2001) *Democratising Globalisation: The Leverage of the Tobin Tax.* London: Zed Books.

Preker, A., Jakab, M. and Schneider, M. (2002) 'Health Financing Reforms in Central and Eastern Europe and the Former Soviet Union', in E. Mossialos, A. Dixon, J. Figueras and J. Kutzin (eds) *Funding Health Care: Options for Europe.* Buckingham: Open University Press.

Rogers, P. (2000) *Losing Control: Global Security in the Twenty-First Century.* London: Pluto Press.

Stockholm International Peace Research Institute (2002) 'Suppliers of Major Conventional Weapons 1996–2000', http://first.sipri.org/index (accessed 2 April).

UNDP (1997) *Ukraine Human Development Report.* Kiev: UNDP.

UNDP (1999a) *Human Development Report for Central and East Europe and the CIS.* UNDP.

UNDP (1999b) *Ukraine Human Development Report.* www.un.kiev.ua:8081/hdr2000. htm.

Wade, R. (2001) *'Is Globalization Making World Income Distribution More Equal?'* LSE-Destin Working Paper No. 01-01. London: LSE.

Woods, N. (2001) 'Order, Globalisation and Inequality in World Politics', in D. Held and A. McGrew (eds) *The Global Transformations Reader.* Cambridge: Polity Press.

World Bank (1993a) *World Development Report: Investing in Health.* Oxford: Oxford University Press.

World Bank (1993b) *Ukraine: The Social Sectors during Transition.* Oxford: World Bank.

World Bank (1996) *World Development Report: From Plan to Market.* Oxford: Oxford University Press.

World Bank (2000) *Country Assistance Evaluation (CAE) 1992–8.* World Bank.

World Bank (2001a) *Ukraine – Social Safety Nets and Poverty.* World Bank.

World Bank (2001b) *World Development Report 2000/2001: Attacking Poverty.* Oxford: Oxford University Press.

World Health Organization (1998) *Health 21.* Geneva: WHO.

World Health Organization (2000a) *The World Health Report 2000. Health Systems: Improving Performance.* Geneva: WHO.

World Health Organization (2000b) *Highlights on Health in Ukraine.* Copenhagen: WHO Regional Office for Europe.

World Health Organization Regional Office for Europe (1985) *Targets for Health For All.* Copenhagen: WHO.

Yergin, D. and Stanislaw, J. (1998) *The Commanding Heights: The Battle between Government and the Marketplace that is Remaking the Modern World.* New York: Simon and Schuster.

Chapter 9

Understanding workplace health promotion

Programme development and evaluation for the small business sector

Lindsey Dugdill

Workplace health promotion: the national and international context

This chapter explores the nature of work and health issues in the small and micro organisation (SME); the process of engaging with and researching businesses; and the practical steps that can be taken to establish collaborative infrastructures for health at work. The content of the chapter draws on research case studies from Merseyside.

Increasing levels of prosperity in Western industrialised nations have not been matched by concomitant health improvement, suggesting the relationship between health and work to be a complex one (Karasek and Theorell 1990). Traditionally, within the UK, workplace health has been viewed as a biomedical issue (for example, an employee accessing the services of an occupational health doctor), or as a health and safety issue (for example, providing safe working conditions for employees). However, important international research (Karasek and Theorell 1990) identified the psychosocial environment as the most influential factor in self-reported ill health among employees; but so far this issue had been neglected within the arena of workplace health promotion. Traditional workplace health provision had often failed to identify the true health needs of employees and consequently health intervention was often inappropriate or too late to prevent long-term absenteeism. Where health provision was available for workers (usually in the larger organisations) it was often provided on a reactive rather than a proactive basis and tended to treat the symptoms rather than the causes of organisational ill health. The interventions and programmes provided often lacked coherence and co-ordination across the institution concerned, and health promotion was seen as a bonus for the workers, rather than a necessity.

In the early 1990s, investigating workers' perceptions of health at work was not deemed a priority and few health intervention programmes in the UK workplace were being systematically measured for effectiveness (Dugdill and Springett 1994). Workplace health programmes were being put in place with no underlying structure of needs assessment and evaluation – hence, the evidence-base for advocating the development of the field of workplace health provision was poor. Also, health practitioners often lacked confidence in being skilled enough to evaluate programmes themselves, thus giving evaluation an aura of mystique and difficulty (personal communication).

Across Europe the nature of work has also been changing dramatically, providing new health challenges – increasingly workers are located within small and medium sized enterprises (SMEs) with no recognised infrastructure of health support. For instance, over half of the UK workforce is employed within an organisation of less than 100 employees (Kavanagh *et al.* 1998). Such businesses survive under extreme financial constraints and hence gaining their interest in and commitment to health promotion is even more difficult. More women have been gaining paid work (39 per cent of EC workforce) leading to changes in the way work is organised; for example, full-time employment is on the decrease, while flexible working patterns are on the increase. The trend is towards less secure working arrangements with many workers being employed on short-term or part-time contracts. All of these factors show the nature of work to be increasingly dynamic, but with a fragmented process and structure likely to bring associated health risk and extreme challenges for the health promoter. Tackling traditional organisations, which have a fairly static workforce and which work between the hours of 'nine-to-five', has been difficult enough. Now, trying to establish good workplace health practice among work structures that are ever changing seems an almost impossible task.

Data on the scale of ill health due to work has been scarce until relatively recently, so its economic impact was not realised. Consequently 'health at work' was fairly low on the political agenda until the beginning of the last decade, when, increasingly, the political and economic importance of the workplace began to be recognised. The documented effectiveness of workplace health interventions in the United States was prompting UK health policy makers to take the subject of workplace health promotion more seriously. This was exemplified by the Conservative government (Department of Health [DoH] 1993), which convened the UK Workplace Taskforce – a multidisciplinary group of professionals, with experience in the field of workplace health. This action was the UK government's strategic response to the improvement of health in the workplace setting, highlighted as a priority target in the *Health of the Nation* strategy (Department of Health [DoH] 1992). The main aims of the Taskforce were to review and assess past and current workplace activity and to advise on the development of activity on health promotion in the workplace. Their development work focused in two particular areas: more effective evaluation of workplace health activity and the marketing of health promotion, particularly among SMEs.

Further surveys in the mid-1990s increased attention on the topic of workplace health. For instance, the Health and Safety Executive (1994) provided evidence to show that each of the 1.5 million workers in the UK with work-related illness cost their employer £400 to £500 per year. In 1998, Tessa Jowell, Minister for Public Health, stated that workplace ill health was costing the country £12 billion, or over £12,000 for every company in the country (Kavanagh *et al.* 1998). The Labour government placed the workplace setting higher on the health agenda by including it within their health strategy *Our Healthier Nation: A Contract for Health* (Department of Health [DoH] 1998).

There is now overwhelming evidence to show that different types of workplace health programmes can lead to economic gains for the organisation involved and probably such evidence is starting to awaken the interest of politicians. Potentially, the main economic benefits of workplace health promotion programmes come about by a reduction in staff turnover, absenteeism rates, accident/injury rates and recruitment costs and/or improvement in corporate image, productivity and risk management (Dugdill and Springett 1994). Considerable evidence exists, especially in the United States, of the economic impact of health promotion programmes in the workplace. For example, a large study with the Du Pont corporation showed that health promotion programmes could reduce absenteeism by 14 per cent with a cost-benefit ratio of $2 saved for every $1 spent on the intervention programme (Bertera 1990). In the UK, there is a growing body of evidence as to the benefits of workplace health promotion, for example the reduction in stress levels reported by ICI-Zeneca employees who participated in a programme of stress management workshops during the early 1990s. There was a general trend for self-reported stress levels to decrease after employees had attended the workshops (Teasdale and McKeown 1994). Recently, the Nuffield Trust (Williams *et al.* 1998) reported on the potential cost saving of reducing absenteeism in the NHS, by only 1 per cent per annum, being as much as £140 million per year.

However, for the small business sector there is very little evidence to substantiate the pattern of benefit illustrated above for large organisations. Nevertheless, recent work carried out on Merseyside has shown economic benefits for SMEs in the following areas: reduction in insurance costs for a construction company that had undertaken safety training; improved competitiveness when bidding for contracts of work for organisations with up-to-date health and safety policies; improved morale leading to improved work performance (Dugdill *et al.* 2000). Supporting evidence for the foregoing is discussed in more detail later on in the chapter.

Repositioning workplace health promotion and evaluation

At a European level the World Health Organization have been leading the field of workplace health promotion for the last decade and Erio Ziglio (Regional Adviser for Health Promotion and Investment, WHO) stated:

The time is ripe for broadening approaches to health promotion research at the work site, which tends to be mainly based on health education only and focus on single health-related subjects. Given the fast changing environment within which public and private companies operate, twenty-first-century health promotion research has to be able to bridge between workplace, family and surrounding community needs and assets for health. The impact of the world of work on social capital, social cohesion and human development in general should and must be directed in a way in which it brings about equitable, sustainable development and health outcome.

(cited in Springett and Dugdill 1999: 5)

This paragraph summarises the importance of workplace health promotion, the need to strive for new ways of understanding health needs and measuring the impact of workplace health programmes, as detailed below. It is argued here that the future for workplace health promotion provision requires a widening of some current approaches being used, and the application of broader, more holistic, models of health than are currently evidenced in the literature. Workers are able to articulate a complex understanding of workplace health issues (Dugdill 2000) and the health programmes provided must begin to reflect that complexity if we are to see an improvement in health gains. This appeal for holistic approaches is not revolutionary (Baric 1990). However, its transfer into practice (in terms of workplace programme design) has been slow, and few well-documented examples exist in the UK literature, particularly of studies following a participatory action research paradigm.

Models of health are numerous (Collins 1997), but their application to the workplace setting are less common. Even today, comprehensive workplace health promotion programmes are rare and are not practised as mainstream business activities. Indeed, it is clear that for many organisations, especially small and medium sized enterprises, health is not considered as an integral part of business management systems (Dugdill et al. 2000). Keeping a business afloat economically is a far higher priority, for most, than implementing policies and support structures for health, and making the economic case for workplace health is a relatively recent phenomenon (Health and Safety Executive [HSE] 1998). Larger organisations, which do have provision for health in terms of occupational, environmental and possibly health promotion services, often do not co-ordinate these services to provide a comprehensive support mechanism for staff that permeates throughout the organisation (personal communication, large petrochemical company, North West England). In general then, the current provision for workplace health promotion in the UK might, at best, be described as heterogeneous.

At a national level, health organisations in the UK have experienced tensions when deciding on the system boundaries of workplace health programmes. For example, in 1993, the Department of Health was still placing great emphasis on programmes that focused on individual lifestyle issues (weight control, drinking behaviour, etc.), reflecting the Conservative government's political ideology about responsibility for health at that time. Towards the latter half of the decade (1990s), a shift in thinking became apparent and the Health Education Authority was clearly embracing organisational approaches to workplace health. For example, they stated in a recent report on the Health at Work in the NHS research project:

> Until recently, the HEA has placed most emphasis on promoting individual healthy lifestyles in its health at work programme. By contrast staff reported to us that their main concerns about health at work were to do with prevention of harm to physical health and organisational factors – the pressure of work, the pace of organisational change and, most particularly, how that change is managed.
>
> (HEA 1999: 2)

Of all agencies, the Health and Safety Executive has perhaps been the most progressive. During the later half of the decade, their mainstream activities moved away from just focusing in the traditional health and safety field, to embracing the psychosocial areas also (HSE 1999), and lately they have taken up the challenge of provision for SMEs (HSE 2000). By the year 2000, a consensus of opinion was forming in the UK about the relative importance of workplace health and a plethora of strategic reports were launched which made the case for improving workplace health provision. These included *Securing Health Together* (Health and Safety Commission 2000), *Improving Working Lives* (Department of Health 2000) and *Their Health in Your Hands* (Confederation of British Industry 2000). Nationally, the scene is set for the twenty-first century being an exciting time for workplace health development.

Key themes for workplace health development

The following key themes are seen as paramount for improving workplace health:

* health practitioner focus;
* measuring complexity;
* gaining access and engaging organisations;
* politicisation of the process of workplace health;
* defining the nature of the small business.

Health practitioner focus

Until relatively recently (1996 onwards), practitioners have lacked guidance and training in the field of workplace health programme development.

Practical involvement with organisations at a local and national level revealed a theory/practice gap to the author, especially in the area of workplace research and evaluation. Training programmes such as Health at Work in the NHS (1996–1999; see HEA 1997) provided simple guidance for NHS staff who were engaging in workplace health programme development.

Common practice showed questionnaires to be the main choice of research tool for establishing baseline data within the workplace setting (author's personal communications). Although practical, these tools did little to establish lines of communication and real understanding about the context of the worker/workplace environment interface, and certainly did not prepare the organisation for intervention or programme development. Indeed, due to the lack of experience, time and monetary resources, the entire planning phase of workplace health programme development and evaluation was often absent from practice. Practitioners wanted to start by gathering data straight away! This resulted in many workplaces being inadequately assessed (poor response to questionnaires being common) and, consequently, inappropriate and under-utilised interventions being provided, which were of no real benefit to the employee or organisation.

Although action research has been accepted and embraced within management literature on organisational change and learning (Preskill and Torres 1999; Coghlan and Brannick 2001), action-orientated research methodologies were often absent from national guidelines on workplace evaluation. These approaches were not considered to be as rigorous and scientifically valid as experimental, positivistic research designs (Oakley *et al.* 1994). Indeed, authors such as Pelletier (1996) have espoused the importance of including qualitative studies in reviews of effectiveness, and then go on to exclude such studies by the nature of their criteria of measurement rigour (Springett and Dugdill 1999).

Internationally, a few researchers have tried the action-orientated research methodologies. For example, Ritchie (1996) described an in-depth, participatory action research (PAR) case study, set in an industrial, Australian workplace. Her reasons for trying this approach were primarily linked to her disillusionment with traditional mechanisms for health intervention, where programmes favoured managers rather than workers, and were not sufficiently tailored to the health needs of the client group and so, subsequently, were not sustainable over time. The principle reason for the choice of such methodology was to work with particular client groups in order to bring about change, in a manner which gave control of the research situation to the workers themselves. Ritchie highlighted the main challenges as ensuring effective entry into the organisation, getting to know the complexity of the context, gaining trust, and keeping momentum going during the relatively long time-frame of the research process. All of these issues are of major importance to the concluding paragraphs of this critical review.

Measuring complexity

Appropriate research and evaluation methodologies must challenge the conventional approaches advocated for testing intervention effectiveness, and evaluation practice should be the focus rather than just measurement itself (Brodie and Dugdill 1993; Springett and Dugdill 1995, 1999). Shaw concurs with this view on evaluation by stating 'Tests of good evaluation are in terms of fairness, an increased awareness of complexity, and an increased understanding of, and respect for, the values of others' (1999: 67).

Action research frameworks can help to shape evaluation methodology, while realistic and appropriate health and business indicators can help to build the evidence-base required to bring the business community on board. Also, innovative ways of working in the health sphere, such as whole-systems approaches, may start to reorient understanding about health provision within organisations, thereby creating infrastructures of health support which transcend organisational boundaries and lead to collaborative systems of support (Dugdill 2000; Dugdill et al. 2001). This is idealistic, but not impossible, and, as the movement of workers into SMEs continues, this networking approach to provision will be essential if health capacity and economic regeneration are to be realised within community settings. Understanding the nature of work and the problems encountered by workers should be the prime focus, rather than an over-emphasis on the work setting. Whole-systems thinking is not new to the organisational development literature (Stacey 1995), but it has rarely been applied to organisational health practice in the UK (Pratt et al. 1999; Dugdill et al. 2001). Pratt et al. described whole-systems thinking as:

> a radical way of thinking about change in complex situations: a combination of theory and practical methods of working across boundaries. At its simplest level it is a way of thinking about and designing meetings that help people to express their different experiences, to identify possibilities for action and commit to change.
>
> (1999: 3)

The King's Fund, while working on the Health at Work in the NHS research project, acknowledged the importance of considering NHS Trusts as 'open, complex systems which were changing rapidly at all levels – paradigmatic, structural, systems, working practice and contextual' (HEA 1999: p9). The methodology adopted in this HEA study was built around the concept of reflective practice, which shares common principles with the action research framework set out in a paper by Dugdill and Springett (1994). The King's Fund emphasised that one of the main challenges facing researchers of complex systems was to balance the need for in-depth, comprehensive measurement with pragmatic, and appropriate, evaluation approaches. An ideal action research approach to programme development and evaluation is often difficult to achieve. Action-orientated methodology is expensive in terms of researcher time and the level of organisational commitment required, and so far the lack of resources, time and expertise have limited the approaches used in workplace research. The relative importance of these practical barriers is magnified in small businesses which have limited time or monetary resources (Dugdill *et al.* 2000).

Compounding these practical difficulties is the barrier of paradigmatic tradition and control of evaluation design. Conventional research methodologies, practised by disciplines such as occupational psychology, are located within the quantitative, experimental paradigm. Such methodologies are often unsuitable for understanding the complexity and context of the workplace setting and do not lead logically to intervention development (Israel *et al.* 1989). Overcoming discipline/paradigm traditions are major challenges for researchers endeavouring to engage in action research in the workplace. Fryer and Feather stated that:

> Action research may be considered to be research in which a central feature of the research design is the explicit intention to optimise the quality of research information and the system under investigation. Much occupational psychology has, however, been conducted within a unitarist frame of reference which tends to make managerial assumptions about the effectiveness of systems under investigation and to accomplish change by further empowering certain, already powerful, interest groups while further disempowering others
>
> (1994: 230)

Only by allowing all stakeholders a voice will a real picture of the important issues for workplace health emerge, and one of the most important factors in successful workplace research is the manner in which businesses and employees are engaged in the research process.

Gaining access and engaging organisation

Entry into, and engagement with, the workplace community is an underexplored area of workplace health research (Deakins 1996). Some of the important factors to consider are management commitment, stakeholder involvement and the political context (Dugdill *et al.* 2000). Overall, engagement with an organisation takes at least six months to plan, and this phase includes working alongside business intermediaries who can give the researcher important intelligence about the workplace community. Ideally, the researcher is trying to build a collaborative and trusting partnership with the organisation. Overcoming scepticism and hostility is necessary within organisations, as people often fear the concept of being evaluated. Turning the process of workplace programme development and evaluation into something positive, valuable to organisational effectiveness and an integral part of business activity, requires a complete 'mind-shift' in thinking about the topic. Thus this phase of engagement requires careful negotiation and explanation, and the organisation has to be given a central role in the control of evaluation design and implementation.

Politicisation of the process of workplace health

Having an integrated approach to workplace health development is vital for success. This approach should concentrate on both programme development and evaluation practice at the grassroots level, and strategic, political thinking at the top – at a regional and national level (Kavanagh *et al.* 1998). This dualistic development requires an understanding of the context of ongoing political processes, which impinge on the workplace setting under investigation and influence potential funding streams.

A partnership approach is now considered fundamental to future health development work and this may be achieved through such government programmes as Health Action Zones, but only if there is sufficient regional awareness and political backing. Building coherent coalitions for health is not easy when partners could be potentially competing for the same funding streams (Kenworthy and Beaumont 2001). Also, partner agencies need to be receptive to new ideas and ways of thinking about service delivery if change is to be achieved (Dugdill *et al.* 2001). Sometimes the very structures and language used within such coalitions can serve to exclude certain groups from applying for funding. Building partnerships for workplace health requires a detailed understanding of both the local economic climate and business structures (for example, Chambers of Commerce). The need for more people-centred thinking has been advocated by Boswell (1999), who argued that, to achieve sustainable economic success and human potential for health, we have to build successful relationships, between individuals, organisations and communities using the values of co-operation, mutuality and negotiation. Concurring with this concept, Stacey (2001) has described the importance of understanding relationships between people when trying to generate change within organisations. However, the relationships that exist within organisations are often hierarchical and militate against health benefit; true democracy within the workplace setting is quite rare (Semler 1994).

Evaluation in itself is a political process, and effective evaluation practice should include an appraisal of local business and health priorities (stakeholder values). However this often creates (or leads to) an ideological tension. For example, striving for economic development can compromise the health of workers if workload increases. Although basic health and safety provision for workers is required by law (Health and Safety at Work Act 1994), most organisations would not consider it their responsibility to deliver programmes of health support that went beyond this. Therefore, in order to access and engage with organisations, an economic argument often has to take place to convince managers of the benefits of investment in the health of the workforce (Dugdill *et al.* 2000). Consequently, indicators included in the evaluation design often have to address the issue of cost-benefit, particularly in small businesses. The measurement of the cost-benefit of workplace health programmes is extremely complex and few examples are provided in the international literature for SMEs. Katz and Peberdy (1997) argue that the application of economic analysis to health promotion is a phenomenon of the 1990s and consequently few examples exist. Measuring the costs and benefits of health promotion programmes requires an understanding of what is important to the business (for example, reducing insurance costs, winning more contracts, etc.) as well as the employee (for example, reduction in self-reported stress) (Brinner and Reynolds 1999). From a health promotion perspective, it is important to ensure that a balance is maintained between monetary benefits, which can be measured, and health benefits, which may be less tangible but no less important (Katz and Peberdy 1997).

Defining the nature of the small business

Small businesses are themselves diverse and can range from the self-employed consultant or tradesman to a GP practice employing twenty people or a small industrial company with fifty employees. Each will have their specific health priorities and needs. Businesses are normally identified by European classification of size as follows: micro (under 10 employees), small (10–49 employees), medium (50–249 employees), large (250-plus employees) (Curran and Blackburn 2001), although there are some variations on these classifications between studies. At the start of 1998, the Department of Trade and Industry estimated there to be 3.7 million businesses in the UK of which 94.8 per cent were micro businesses and 4.4 per cent were small organisations (Curran and Blackburn 2001) – they form, by far, the majority of all organisations and account for approximately 40 per cent of all employment. Small businesses are vital to economic regeneration, especially in such areas as the industrial North West. The health of employees is therefore paramount in the regeneration process and any infrastructure of support that promotes health and well-being will be contributing to the developing capacity of the area. There is a growing acceptance of this hypothesis, for example Beveridge, stated:

> There is now widespread acceptance of the notion that the creation and growth of small companies is at the heart of the economic development process. In particular, the fact that small businesses have proved much more effective at generating employment than larger firms – and have been

doing for the past twenty or thirty years – has made the development of small businesses of major interest to government, academics, educators and financiers.

(cited in Deakins *et al.* 1997: xi)

Considering the rapid expansion (and economic importance) of the small business sector, it is surprising that so few studies are reported (Dugdill *et al.* 2000), especially concerning personnel and health issues. As highlighted recently by Curran and Blackburn, assumptions are often made about the nature and concerns of SMEs being 'just scaled down versions of larger firms' (2001: 3). However, this is not so, as small businesses report very specific health concerns, such as long working hours, poor physical working environments, economic constraints and pressure on team members when other workers are absent (Dugdill and Coffey 2001). Also, other inequalities exist between large and small organisations, such as lack of a clear infrastructure for health and safety support; lack of representation for workers (no union structure); and health issues not always being seen to be essential to small business practice (health and safety not deemed a necessity for supporting a new business financially). Organisations with less than five employees do not have a legal obligation to have written health and safety policies in place – this in itself can lead to lack of awareness of the importance of employee health, and avoidance of meeting the minimum standards required by law, for example, compulsory breaks, access to fresh drinking water, etc.

In terms of developing workplace health research and intervention programmes with SMEs there are many challenges to be faced, such as acquiring enough trust and confidence to gain access to the business, and dealing with lack of stability of the sector, that is, because there is a dynamic turnover (start-up and closure of businesses), the delivery of support must be flexible. Also, intervention support needs to be practical, low cost and specific to the needs of the business. Traditional delivery of health and safety training, for instance, is often too expensive and not specific enough to the contextual needs of a business. As Curran and Blackburn articulate 'the apparent simplicity of the small business has tripped up a lot of researchers. Small does not mean simple ... indeed, it can be argued that small enterprises are actually more difficult to study than large enterprises' (2001: 4).

There is a need to recognise the dynamic nature of work in the twenty-first century, where the pace of change within organisations is accelerating, so that organisational change is the 'status quo' (Preskill and Torres 1999). However, there are fundamental differences between the different organisational size sectors, with smaller organisations facing the fastest pace of change, but having less money and personnel time to invest in developing support structures for health. Conversely, larger organisations are more likely to have some sort of provision for health (for example, an occupational health service) already in place, but they have other barriers to overcome when trying to bring about positive changes for health, such as hierarchical structures which interfere with communication. Interventions often take longer to put in place within larger organisations due to the slower pace of change. Despite the resource limitations faced by smaller organisations, they have some advantages over larger organisations, in that they can respond more rapidly to health challenges.

Consequently, the emphasis given to the research process and methodology will vary depending on the type, and size of organisation that is being studied. Research methodologies practised within small organisations have to be simple, quick to administer and completely relevant to the business concerned (for example, short group meetings and interviews can work well). Needs identification can be relatively quick if staff numbers are low. Once these businesses are on board it is possible to engage in an action research cycle, although continued access to the organisation has to take place in short bursts of activity that fit in with business priorities such as timing of shift working. Engagement can be prolonged if a trusting relationship between manager and researcher is established and the perception of the benefits of health activity are positive. Time-intensive methodologies such as Open Space events (Pratt *et al.* 1999; Preskill and Torres 1999; Dugdill *et al.* 2001), which are used within whole-systems working, are not practicable unless some form of financial reimbursement or incentive is made available to businesses. The resource limitations within SMEs curtail participation in development and evaluation work. Small organisations are often as responsive to new, creative and innovative ideas as they are used to a risk-taking culture (Deakins 1996), and much can be achieved if organisations come together to support each other on a community basis.

Larger organisations have more time and money to commit to the research process and are more likely to be able to afford to implement new health programmes compared with SMEs. One of the main challenges for the researcher in a large organisation, is to understand the range of issues that are of concern to workers and to facilitate the prioritisation of these issues – there may be a large disparity between managers' and employees' views on health (Dugdill 1996). Some form of workplace questionnaire is often a useful research method, but only when used in association with qualitative methods and after focus groups have first been used to narrow the organisational health agenda (Dugdill 1996, 2001). As with small organisations, the action research process is possible, but only after careful negotiation through senior management and stakeholder commitment. Evaluation feedback is important in organisational development for health. However, it may require more effort to achieve effective feedback in a large organisation, due to the problems of organisational structure and hierarchy.

Researching health within small businesses in Merseyside

The *Health at Work Strategy for Liverpool* (Kavanagh *et al.* 1998) identified some interesting characteristics of the workforce in Merseyside. The number of small companies (0–24 employees) increased by 12.5 per cent between 1987 and 1991, whereas the number of large organisations (500-plus employees) decreased by 21 per cent (compared with 13 per cent nationally); 51 per cent of the workforce were women, 24.3 per cent of whom worked part-time compared with only 4.9 per cent of men who were part-time workers. Self-employment was reported to be below the national average. Overall, there is a picture of increased job flexibility and intermittent employment history, leading to short-term and casual employment. These changes could result in increased risks from occupational ill health. It is against this picture of a dynamically changing workforce that the following research case study was carried out in south Liverpool.

Research case study 1: developing health and safety interventions for small business, Speke/Garston, Liverpool

To explore the health needs of small businesses, an empirical evaluation study was carried out between 1996 and 1998, in a deprived area of south Liverpool, UK (Dugdill *et al.* 2000). The study was designed to evaluate the process and impact of health and safety intervention uptake in small businesses. It was one of the first studies in the UK to document health and economic benefits for the micro sector (businesses with fewer than ten employees) and was, therefore, filling a vital gap in the workplace health promotion literature. Some of the major challenges to workplace health provision are faced by this sector, as the rapid expansion of the small business community across the UK has led to the existence of many unregulated businesses, with little or no health advice or provision for employees. Also, health promotion professionals and enforcement agencies (Environmental Health/Health and Safety Executive), who recognise the needs of these businesses, often do not have the skills or resources to reach them in an appropriate manner, that is, in a way that will encourage and facilitate health actions. The extreme economic constraints faced by SMEs often lead to working practices which are unsafe or unsound in some way, for example, very long working hours, reduction of the amount of time spent on safety procedures, etc. Changing this type of organisational thinking towards health will require the development of an evidence base which provides details of the health and economic benefits to be gained by taking a proactive approach to health at work issues. Three research questions were explored during this study:

1   How was health and safety support for SMEs planned and provided?
2   What was the intervention uptake?
3   What were the perceived benefits of those interventions from the busi-
    nesses' perspective?

The evaluation study attempted to follow an action research paradigm
and was an integral part of the project from inception. As accessing SMEs is
extremely difficult, due to time constraints placed upon businesses, appropriate methodology for the research had to be developed, including a
telephone survey, and in-depth, case study interviews. A range of quantitative and qualitative indicators were incorporated in the study design, for
example, a number of businesses from each sector taking up different types
of intervention (quantitative); perceived benefits of intervention (qualitative). Data was also collected from businesses (n = 140) and key informants
from within the local business community.

Process

The process of setting-up an infrastructure of health and safety provision
was complex. It involved undertaking a detailed six-month consultation
with local businesses, business associations and other service providers in the
area. During the consultation, it emerged that the safety aspect of health
and safety provision was deemed a priority. Four specific interventions were
designed for SMEs:

- a health and safety information pack;
- workplace health and safety inspections;
- health and safety policies for the workplace;
- health and safety training.

Costing and marketing these interventions appropriately were the next
components of the process. The first two interventions were free and the
second two were costed at £40/hour.

Philosophical approach of the project

The project provided health and safety support in a manner which encom-
passed central values of health promotion practice – empowerment and
enablement (Ottawa Charter for Health Promotion 1986). The overall aim
was to work with the local business community, assess the priority health
needs, develop appropriate interventions and evaluate their effectiveness
before feeding the information back to the community involved. This was
achieved with a facilitative action approach that enabled the businesses to
learn how to develop their own health and safety capability rather than rely

on expensive consultant-led support, which has been the normal model of provision. Capacity-building is a key tenet of health and economic regeneration and health promotion practice is about finding the right processes by which to achieve this development. This research study showed that the above facilitative approach was possible and had many perceivable benefits to business. It may be a better way of enabling compliance rather than using the threat of legislative action as in the past.

Intervention uptake

In total 140 businesses contacted the project for health and safety support over eighteen months. Of those, 120 took up one or more of the interventions offered above. The most popular interventions were those offered free of charge; however, construction and manufacturing sectors showed a willingness to pay for the interventions that cost money. This was not a surprising result when you consider the necessity of construction businesses to prove compliance with health and safety legislation. Lower uptake of costed interventions in the retail and service sectors may reflect an inability or unwillingness to pay. It is apparent that in these sectors, where perceived health risk is lower, education may be necessary to encourage businesses to invest in health and safety support.

Perceived benefits

Businesses revealed a variety of perceived benefits via the telephone survey and the in-depth interviews. These benefits included improvement in company image, increased ability to win contracts, lowering of insurance premiums, increased confidence to tackle health and safety issues in the future.

Methodological limitations

A 'portfolio approach' to evaluation was taken with this study, and a range of quantitative and qualitative methods were used in an ongoing, action research model. Certain methods were quite successful at gathering valid data from small businesses – interviews, telephone interviews and group discussions. These methods were only successful because the questions were directly relevant to the business community and were very quick to administer (e.g. 15-minute interviews). Postal surveys (questionnaires) proved to be ineffective as a research method and elicited a very low response rate. Using business intermediaries to access the business community also proved invaluable to the research process. Ongoing engagement in the research process was possible once businesses gained trust in the researcher.

This study showed that participatory mechanisms of intervention development and evaluation can be employed if used sensitively. The study showed that health interventions would be accessed by small businesses if supplied within a cost-effective and trustworthy system of support.

Research case study 2: health at work consultation exercise, Sefton, Merseyside

The following information is taken from a detailed health at work consultation exercise carried out across the borough of Sefton, Merseyside, during 2000–1 (Dugdill and Coffey 2001), and which was commissioned by Sefton Strategic Health at Work Partnership.

Sefton has an extensive mix of employment and business organisations, with approximately 83,600 employees in total working within 7,995 units (Annual Employment Survey 1997). The national trend towards increasing employment in SMEs is matched within Sefton where 52.1 per cent of the employed population work in a business with less than 50 employees; 82.8 per cent of business organisations (units) fall into the micro sector. Again, this data corroborates the pattern of employment seen across the Merseyside region (Kavanagh *et al.* 1998). The predominant sectors in Sefton in terms of employment are public administration, distribution/ hotels, banking/finance, and manufacturing.

The borough of Sefton is heterogeneous with a relatively affluent, ageing population, living in the north sector (encompassing Southport). This is an area predominated by consumer and tourist industries and flanked by agriculture. This is in contrast to the southern part of the borough, which is exemplified by pockets of extreme deprivation and unemployment (Bootle). Historically, the latter is a dockland area which has provided a work infrastructure for south Sefton, but again a shift to employment within SMEs is seen. A few large employers are also located in Bootle, for example, the Health and Safety Executive, the Inland Revenue and insurance companies such as the Alliance & Leicester.

Table 9.1   Employment in Sefton by size of unit (1997)

Number of Employees	Employees by size of unit: 1997 (NOMIS)	
	Emps	%
1–10	19,000	22.7
11–49	24,600	29.4
50–199	21,000	25.2
200+	19,000	22.7
Total	83,600	100.0

Note: NOMIS employment figures are rounded off to the nearest 100 to comply with regulations.

Table 9.2   Units in Sefton by sizeband (1997)

Number of employees	Units	%
1–10	6,617	82.8
11–49	1,120	14.0
50–199	222	2.8
200+	36	0.5
Total	7,995	100.0

Source: Annual Employment Survey, Office for National
Statistics (NOMIS).

The consultation was used to gather baseline information about health, safety and welfare at work issues across the borough. It was also an awareness-raising exercise in terms of providing information about the Health at Work strategy development and existing support services. The research process was designed to be sensitive to economic and business priorities and the following research questions served as a framework for information collection.

1   What are the existing health, safety, and welfare problems within work-places from different sectors?
2   What are the main causes of absenteeism? What could reduce this? How do you finance it?
3   What provision is currently made within your organisation to support the health of employees?
4   What information would be useful to you in enabling you to support the health of employees?
5   What are the priority areas for intervention action?
6   What methods could help to support these actions?
7   What types of Partnerships/external support could help to achieve improved health at work?

The consultation comprised of stakeholder interviews and a large postal survey of organisations, from the public, private and voluntary sectors. The survey was unique in both its size (n = 203) and the number of respondents from the small and micro sector (n = 169). The key aims of the consultation were to assess current health, safety and welfare priorities across sectors, current provision for health at work, areas for action and intervention development, barriers preventing development and potential solutions to those barriers.

Comparison across sectors

The main findings were that health at work activity was most prevalent in the areas of health and safety, sickness/absenteeism management, smoking policy and manual handling. Areas where policy was less likely to be developed included anti-bullying, childcare and family-friendly practice. Large organisations, particularly in the public and voluntary sector, were more likely to report ill health, low morale and absenteeism problems when compared with the small, micro and private sectors. Also, large organisations tended to exhibit psychosocial problems of poor communication, lack of support networks and poor management practice, which was probably contributing to the stress reported. Small business, on the other hand, cited the physical working environment as the main factor affecting health of employees. Stress in this sector was caused by workload, meeting deadlines and the state of the economic climate, as exemplified in this quote: 'Workload is the main cause of stress because we are a small business increasing in size more rapidly than we expected' (manufacturing business 20–49 employees).

Overwhelmingly, the area of workplace health that most organisations (irrespective of size or sector) wanted to develop was around stress management. Other areas for improvement included family-friendly policies, workload and job content. The key barriers to workplace health activity were lack of monetary resources, having the expertise/skills, and having 'too much change to keep up with'. Support was most commonly requested in the areas of advice giving, monetary resources (grants), training, and free health and safety checks.

Small and micro business priorities: why health is important to the organisation

The following quotes explain the meaning of health to small business.

Without our employees our business cannot function to the best of its ability. (Caravan park, 50–99 employees)

It is important that our staff feel safe and well looked after so that their work performance is not affected by ill health or injury. (Transport sector, 50–99 employees)

Reflects on behaviour towards customers. (Retail sector, self-employed)

It won't function without health. (Public administration, sole trader)

Small and micro business priorities

The policies most likely to be already in place were health and safety, sickness/absence, and smoking. The policies that this sector wanted to develop were stress management, family-friendly, and health and safety. They also wanted to improve the physical working environment. Barriers to implementing change for health at work were resources (time/money), having the skills and expertise and knowing which issues were priorities. Approximately 80 per cent saw workplace health as the responsibility of workers and/or businesses alone – and not a collective responsibility involving other agencies.

Consultation recommendations

The recommendations arising out of this research were:

1   to raise awareness of the infrastructure for health at work activity in Sefton, and provide advice and information;
2   to provide appropriate support for business and organisations in a format that is accessible to them;
3   to prioritise interventions such as stress management, improving the physical and psychosocial work environment, and developing family-friendly policies;
4   to co-ordinate the infrastructure for health at work through the Sefton Strategic Health at Work Partnership;
5   to develop the evidence base for health at work practice;
6   to share good practice through exemplar organisations and establishing minimum standards;
7   to develop a full action plan for health at work activity aimed at all sectors across Sefton, that enables capacity-building within business and organisations.

Conclusion

The approaches advocated above for workplace health programme development and evaluation, are both collective and participatory (Libertarian/ Radical), as described by Beattie (1993). Central features of the approach are action research methodology, development and sharing of skills, increasing political awareness for workplace health and community development. The author goes further, to suggest that whole-systems thinking could introduce a new dimension to workplace development and evaluation, but only if applied in a practical way (Dugdill *et al.* 2001). The main emphasis is on the importance of appropriate engagement with organisations and the rigorous practice of intervention design and evaluation.

The need to focus workplace health research attention on small and micro businesses has recently been highlighted by the European Foundation for the Improvement of Living and Working Conditions (1999), which recognised the dearth of evidence in this sector. In the future, workplaces will consist of fewer large organisations (with rigid structures and hierarchies) and more small companies (with shorter life trajectories and flatter structures). Consequently, there will be a need for a multi-skilled workforce who are prepared to take short-term contracts and to move between jobs more often. Also, rapid development of information technology has enabled workers to be more mobile and to work in different places. Thus it appears that what is needed in the future for workplace health development are flexible structures and approaches that reflect the dynamic nature of work: transferring skills for health improvement to people who can take them with them when they move jobs, and research that explores the mechanisms which impact on health in the workplace setting. Every workplace setting has a unique context so, although the practice of evaluation can be transferable, each workplace setting/community needs to be considered individually. There is a need to move away from traditional approaches to evaluation and to use techniques which have meaning within the setting concerned such as image-based or IT-based evaluation (Mann and Stewart 2000; Dugdill 2001) and methods which can allow ongoing exploration and development within the workplace/community setting. Sharing of health provision across organisations will be much more cost-effective than having replicated services within each workplace. Local outreach workers can provide health expertise at a low or subsidised cost, and in a confidential and supportive manner, and build local skill-based capacity. A recognition of the importance of building relationships, skills and good intervention and evaluation practice are of paramount importance to the future of workplace health promotion.

Acknowledgements

The author would like to thank the collaborative contributions of Liverpool Occupational Health Partnership, Sefton Strategic Health at Work Partnership and all the organisations and employees who took part in the research.

References

Baric, L. (1990) 'A Healthy Enterprise in a Healthy Environment', *Journal for the Institute of Health Education* 28(3): 84–91.

Beattie, A. (1993) 'The Changing Boundaries of Health', in A. Beattie, M. Gott, L. Jones, M. Sidell (eds) *Health and Wellbeing: A Reader*. Basingstoke: Oxford University Press/Macmillan.

Bertera, R.L. (1990) 'The Effects of Health Promotion on Absenteeism and Employment Costs in a Large Industrial Population', *American Journal of Public Health* 80(9): 1101–5.

Boswell, J. (1999) *Community and the Economy: The Theory of Public Cooperation*. London: Routledge.

Brinner, R.B. and Reynolds, S. (1999) 'The Costs, Benefits and Limitations of Organisational Level Stress Interventions', *Journal of Organisational Behaviour* 20: 647–64.

Brodie, D. and Dugdill, L. (1993) 'Health Promotion at Work', *Journal of the Royal Society of Medicine* 86: 694–6.

Coghlan, D. and Brannick, T. (2001) *Doing Action Research in Your Own Organisation*. London: Sage.

Collins, T. (1997) 'Models of Health: Pervasive, Persuasive and Politically Charged', in M. Sidell, L. Jones, J. Katz and A. Peberdy (eds) *Debates and Dilemmas in Promoting Health*. Basingstoke: OUP/Macmillan.

Confederation of British Industry (2000) *Their Health in your Hands: Focus on Occupational Partnerships*. Waterside Press.

Curran, J. and Blackburn, R.A. (2001) *Researching the Small Enterprise*. London: Sage.

Deakins, D. (1996) *Entrepreneurship and Small Firms*. London: McGraw-Hill.

Deakins, D., Jennings, P. and Mason, C. (1997) *Small Firms: Entrepreneurship and the Nineties*. London: Paul Chapman Publishing.

Department of Health (DoH) (1992) *Health of the Nation*. London: DoH.

Department of Health (DoH) (1993) *The Health of the Nation: Workplace Task Force Report*. London: DoH.

Department of Health (DoH) (1998) *Our Healthier Nation: A Contract for Health*. London: DoH.

Department of Health (DoH) (2000) *Improving Working Lives Standard*. London: DoH.

Dugdill, L. (1996) *NHS Staff Needs Assessment: A Practical Guide*. London: Health Education Authority.

Dugdill, L. (2000) 'Developing a Holistic Understanding of Workplace Health: The Case of Bankworkers', *Ergonomics* 43(10): 1738–49.

Dugdill, L. (2001) *Framework for Action Supplement: Guidance on Evaluation*. London: Health Education Authority.

Dugdill, L. and Coffey, M. (2001) *Their Health: Our Wealth*. Sefton Health Authority: Sefton Health at Work Consultation Report.

Dugdill, L. and Springett, J. (1994) 'Evaluation of Workplace Health Promotion: A Review', *Health Education Journal* 53: 337–47.

Dugdill, L., James, K., Cliff, E. and Powell, E. (2001) *Developing Whole Systems: Theory to Practice*. Liverpool: Liverpool Community Health Council.

Dugdill, L., Kavanagh, C., Barlow, J., Nevin, I. and Platt, G. (2000) 'The Development and Uptake of Health and Safety Interventions Aimed at Small Businesses', *Health Education Journal* 59: 157–65.

European Foundation for the Improvement of Living and Working Conditions (1999) *New Approaches to Improve the Health of a Changing Workforce*. Luxembourg: Office for Official Publications of the European Communities.

Fryer, D. and Feather, N.T. (1994) 'Intervention Techniques', in C. Cassell and G. Symon (eds) *Qualitative Methods in Organisational Research: A Practical Guide*. London: Sage.

Health and Safety Commission (HSC) (2000) *Securing Health Together*. London: HSC.

Health and Safety Executive (HSE) (1994) *The Cost to the British Economy of Work Accidents and Work-related Ill Health*. London: HSE.

Health and Safety Executive (HSE) (1998) *Developing an Occupational Health Strategy for Great Britain*. Norwich: HMSO.

Health and Safety Executive (HSE) (1999) *Guidelines for HSE's Research Programmes*. Norwich: HMSO.

Health and Safety Executive (HSE) (2000) *An Evaluation of the Safety Information Centre Approach in Providing Health and Safety Advice to Small Firms*. Norwich: HMSO.

Health Education Authority (HEA) (1997) *Making the Case for Health at Work in the NHS: Briefing Pack*. London: HEA.

Health Education Authority (HEA) (1999) *Up the Down Escalator?* London: HEA.

Israel, B., Schurman, S.J. and House, J.S. (1989) 'Action Research on Occupational Stress: Involving Researchers', *International Journal of Health Services* 19(1): 135–55.

Karasek, R. and Theorell, T. (1990) *Healthy Work: Stress, Productivity and the Reconstruction of Working Life*. New York: Basic Books.

Katz, J. and Peberdy, A. (eds) (1997) *Promoting Health: Knowledge and Practice*. Basingstoke: OUP/Macmillan.

Kavanagh, C., Barlow, J. and Dugdill, L. (1998) *Health at Work Strategy for Liverpool*. Liverpool: Liverpool Occupational Health Project.

Kenworthy, A. and Beaumont, S. (2001) *Health Improvement and Health Inequalities in Merseyside – Taking stock of the Merseyside Health Action Zone*. District Audit for the Audit Commission.

Mann, C. and Stewart, F. (2000) *Internet Communication and Qualitative Research: A Handbook for Researching Online*. London: Sage.

Oakley, A., France-Dawson, M. and Holland, J. (1994) *Workplace Interventions – Does Health Promotion Work?* London: Health Education Authority.

Pelletier, K.R. (1996) 'A Review and Analysis of the Health and Cost-Effective Outcome Studies of Comprehensive Health Promotion and Disease Prevention Programmes at the Work Site: 1991–1993 update', *American Journal of Health Promotion* 8: 50–62.

Pratt, J., Gordon, P. and Plamping, D. (1999) *Working Whole Systems: Putting Theory into Practice in Organisations*. London: King's Fund Publishing.

Preskill, H. and Torres, R.T. (1999) *Evaluative Enquiry for Learning in Organisations*. London: Sage.

Ritchie, J.E. (1996) 'Using Participatory Research to Enhance Health in the Work Setting: An Australian Experience', in K. de Koning and M. Martin (eds) *Participatory Research in Health: Issues and Experiences*. London: Zed Books.

Semler, R. (1994) *Maverick: The Story Behind the World's Most Unusual Workplace*. London: Arrow Books.

Shaw, I.F. (1999) *Qualitative Evaluation*. London: Sage.

Springett, J. and Dugdill, L. (1995) 'Workplace Health Promotion Programmes: Towards a Framework for Evaluation', *Health Education Journal* 54: 88–98.

Springett, J. and Dugdill, L. (1999) *Health Promotion Policies and Programmes in the Workplace: A New Challenge for Evaluation*, European Health Promotion Series No. 7. Copenhagen: World Health Organisation/EURO.

Stacey, R. (1995) 'Creativity in Organisations: The Importance of Mess', Professorial Lecture Series, University of Hertfordshire.

Stacey, R. (2001) *Complex Responsive Processes in Organisations: Learning and Knowledge Creation*. London: Routledge.

Teasdale, E.L. and McKeown, S. (1994) 'Managing Stress at Work: The ICI-Zeneca Pharmaceuticals Experience 1986–1993', in C.L. Cooper and S. Williams (eds) *Creating Healthy Work Organisations*. Chichester: John Wiley.

Williams, S., Michie, S. and Pattani, S. (1998) *Improving the Health of the NHS Workforce*. London: The Nuffield Trust.

World Health Organization (1986) 'Ottawa Charter for Health Promotion', *Journal of Health Promotion* 1: 1–4.

Chapter 10

Health promotion and alternative medicine

Linda Gibson

Drawing on interviews undertaken for an ethnographic study of professionalisation and alternative medicine in the UK, this chapter explores accounts from alternative practitioners about the kind of health work that they do. What struck me during the research was that, in describing the work they do, key concepts used in the promotion of health discourse were mirrored, and it is this I want to explore. By doing so I hope to draw some conclusions on the implications of a congruency, or 'fit', between them for both policy and practice of alternative medicine and health promotion. For alternative medicine, there are key implications arising from the debate about the integration of therapies into mainstream health services, which are currently dominated, at public level, by medicine. This debate focuses on developing the evidence for alternative medicine and extracting techniques, using what 'works', to deal with symptoms and pathology. However, if the work of alternative medicine mirrors a salutogenic, health-promoting perspective of health, as I suggest, harnessing this may provide an opportunity to reorientate and move forward a public health agenda that is able to provide a community-based network of health delivery that is inclusive, equitable and driven from the grassroots.

The research was an ethnography on the effects of professionalisation on three particular therapies – osteopathy, aromatherapy and reflexology – chosen because they represented different stages of the process. The implementation of strategies of professionalisation – such as regulation, registration and standardisation – on the different therapies, was demonstrated, in the study, to draw on and replicate traditional public gendered roles. From this perspective, the work of alternative medicine is expressed as a function of feminised caring and communication skills, such as touch and time. However, the national debates focus on technical aspects, such as the need to develop a critical mass of evidence for incorporation into the NHS. Certain therapies, such as homeopathy, herbalism, acupuncture and osteopathy, jostle in a hierarchy of medical acceptability, while others are relegated to the irrational, 'woolly' end of the spectrum. Meanwhile, the interviews with practitioners revealed that the everyday praxis of alternative medicine retains its core tenets of holism and vitalism. These were embedded in a coherent philosophical model of health that focused on well-being, empowerment and healing, a discourse increasingly underpinning health promotion. In reality, many practitioners were practising a number of therapeutic modalities, rather than the one I had identified them with. They articulated their practice as unified and integrative, bringing together the personal and the social in the therapeutic encounter. Many of these practitioners were engaged in flexible, part-time work within the private sector (their own/joint private practice), the voluntary /non-statutory sectors and, to a lesser degree, the statutory sector (predominantly at primary care level). Many of the practitioners were working part time with local, innovative, community projects, funded and run through local healthy public policy initiatives such Health Action Zones (HAZ), Healthy Living Centres, and Sure Start projects, aimed at reducing inequalities in health. Much of this work was performed by the practitioners at an informal and voluntary (i.e. unpaid) level. Debates about the potential gains and losses of this sort of work for therapists, and about conditions of service, are still to be articulated (Donnelly 2001). However, this move in policy towards placing partnership working at the centre of current health and social care reforms (Department of Health [DoH] 1999) suggests a shift towards a social model of care. Underpinned by the 1999 Health Act this partnership working is seen as a way of stimulating collaboration between agencies (rather than the competitive market-driven services) and establishing opportunities for key stakeholders to shape services. Health promotion is increasingly characterised by working with key stakeholders or agents in decision making processes that affect outcomes (Springett 2001), although the means of achieving collaborative practice are still not fully understood. Working with people and communities, 'people-centred health promotion' (Raeburn and Rootman 1998) requires an ecological and holistic approach to health, one that can capture complex social phenomena (Springett 2001). Within health promotion, key principles of sustainability and community development are focused on. My research uncovered an informal network of alternative practitioners working in settings that reflect these aims. Harnessing that work in a collaborative manner would provide a means for achieving such an agenda.

Alternative medicine

The use and practice of alternative medicine is now widespread throughout Britain, North America and Europe (MORI 1989; Emslie *et al.* 1996; Kelner and Wellman 1997) and it has grown, in the UK, to provide a substantial subsidiary healthcare system (Fulder 1996). One in four people in the UK say they use alternative medicine, with the figure doubling during the 1990s (Mills and Peacock 1997). Other surveys suggest that up to 20 per cent of the population in the UK have been treated by complementary and alternative medicine (CAM) (Ernst and White 2000). Implicit in this growth of use is an increase in practitioner numbers also (Mills and Budd, 2000), although studies of this increase tend to measure official membership of practitioner organisations of the most recognisable therapies, ignoring the broad scope of the informal sector, where the use and practice of alternative medicine is substantial but may be less open to surveillance. What this suggests is that alternative medicine is now an established pattern of care alongside other models of health such as biomedical, folk and lay systems. Scrambler argues that this rise in the use of, and interest in, alternative medicine gives Kleinman's original 'folk' sector thesis '*a new salience*' (2002: 111). The rise of the consumer-driven market in people's choice of healthcare is also seen as important (Coward 1989; Bakx 1991; Fulder 1996). This 'consumer-led boom' (Dickenson 1996:150) has, over the last twenty years, utilised alternative medicine to express its dissatisfaction with both doctors (Furnham and Bhagrath 1993; Vincent *et al.* 1995) and NHS service provision. Users of therapies are pragmatic, using them alongside conventional care (Sharma 1995). The 'smart consumer' (Kelner and Wellman 1997) can be identified as a well-informed individual who will choose specific practitioners for specific complaints according to personal preference or recommendation.

Public demand for alternative therapies has forced allopathic medicine to pay them more attention and, increasingly, certain therapies are being integrated within parts of the NHS, but perhaps more particularly, and successfully, within primary healthcare (Pietroni 1990), the Hospice movement (Morris 1996) and oncology units. A report by the NHS Confederation found:

> a gradual introduction of CM (Complementary Medicine) at 'grass roots' level in the NHS, across the range of healthcare professionals. It appears that, as CM becomes increasingly used, it is gradually accepted into mainstream practice.
>
> (1997: 2)

The recent House of Lords *Sixth Report on Complementary and Alternative Medicine* (2000) recommended that universities and the Royal Colleges should familiarise their medical students, doctors, dentists and veterinary surgeons with CAM, so that they could provide information to their patients and retain their gatekeeping role (Owen *et al.* 2001), an important professional function. However, it would appear that certain therapies are more acceptable for integration into mainstream practice than others, and there are concerns that therapies which are embedded within traditional or indigenous healing systems are being excluded from the debates (Stone 2001). For example, in the aforementioned House of Lords report (2000) Ayurvedic medicine and traditional Chinese medicine were left out because 'there is no established evidence supporting these'. Organisations such as the Foundation for Integrated Medicine (FIM) provide some practitioners and their professional bodies with forums and practical assistance in examining and setting up regulatory processes (FIM 2002). FIM, along with other bodies, believes that the legal and regulatory mechanisms of medicine may not be appropriate for many therapies, which claim differing epistemological roots. Increasingly, a mechanism of voluntary self-regulation is perceived as the most appropriate for most therapies (Stone and Matthews 1995; Mills and Budd 2000). However, I would suggest that the public rhetoric of integration of alternative medicine into mainstream healthcare delivery continues to be dominated by a powerful medical lobby, which attempts to define the parameters of regulation and practice (Stone and Matthews 1996) and leads the call for therapies to be evaluated for their clinical effectiveness and for the investigation of their 'scientific basis'. While this is important, this genre of research tends to draw on narrow definitions of evidence, focusing only on specific pathology, symptoms and aetiology, as demonstrated in the Royal London Homeopathic Hospital's Report (RLHH 1999). Traditional, scientific methods such as the randomised controlled trial (RCT) (Ernst 1996; Vickers *et al.* 1997) and 'rational evidence-based' research (RLHH 1999) are advocated, paralleling the current drive for evidence-based medicine (EBM). Other methods, drawn from social sciences, are consequently assigned to the 'woolly', or 'soft' data bin, although there is some evidence of action research approaches being applied, particularly in primary care. Consequently, integration can be seen as selecting certain therapies for their (proven) techniques for adding into the medical repertoire:

> these innovative *techniques* [my emphasis] should be rigorously assessed and, where appropriate, integrated into mainstream conventional medicine.
>
> (House of Lords 2000)

All of this leads me to assert that incorporation, or even assimilation, rather than integration is the political agenda, and to agree with Saks's (2000) assertion that it is the professional self-interests of medicine that lie behind moves to import therapies into the NHS.

However, on the more positive side, I would argue that, along with other factors, alternative medicine *is* effecting changes in the institution of medicine, forcing it to become more responsive and reflexive. Medical schools are increasingly using alternative medicine as a way of getting students to reflect on their practice as future doctors. A module on 'Human Healing' at Glasgow University provides a good example of this. Medical students reported being encouraged to see 'a bigger picture' in terms of human and therapeutic interactions, broadening their perceptions of health and healing, and challenging their orthodox scientific training (Bryden 1999). Doctors who undertake training in alternative medicine appear to report a number of benefits, such as the opportunity to engage their feelings, (re)-discover their intuitive skills and enjoy therapeutic touch (Owen *et al.* 2001), although the adequacy of such training for healthcare professionals is a contentious issue in itself. How deeply these changes are impacting on medicine is difficult to say at this stage.

While the medical debate tends to focus on the more visible, or 'legitimate' therapies, or those that have been more successful in coalescing, such as osteopathy, herbalism, acupuncture or reflexology, many therapists in these and other fields, operate in the more informal, folk sector. These practitioners prefer to work at a more local, community-based level. The majority of alternative therapies are drawn from a model underpinned by vitalism. Vitalistic or energy-based theories continue to be rejected because they do not fit conventional, scientific orthodoxy (Benor 1995). The mechanisms of such therapies are reduced to their purely physiological effects, as demonstrated in the case of acupuncture (Saks 1991; Scheid 1993) and osteopathy. Claims of vitalism are quietly put aside for acceptance by allopathy, as in the case of the successful bid for regulation by the osteopaths; and other therapies such as aromatherapy and reflexology are perceived as so non-invasive that they pose little risk or indeed challenge. The problem this raises is that alternative medicine is then incorporated into mainstream healthcare delivery, losing its radical potential for enlarging our view of health and wellness. The very success of alternative medicine in the public arena neutralises its paradigmatic challenge. Defining health differently from the dominant discourse of biomedicine, an alternative perspective draws historically on folk definitions such as the 'will to be well' and 'well-being' models (Fulder 1995: 23). Health promotion, however, appears to provide a model for the integration of alternative medicine that is consistent with the latter's central tenets. The promotion of health and well-being is central to the praxis of alternative medicine. Surprisingly, perhaps, the links between the two are still to be theorised, although there are some notable exceptions (Braathen 1996; Goldstein 2000).

Interviews with alternative practitioners

As in any emerging discipline, terminology and the use of language becomes subject to powerful political processes. Various terms have been used and are reflected in the literature: complementary medicine, complementary and alternative medicine (CAM), integrated medicine (the current favourite), traditional, non-orthodox or vibrational. These are not by any means exhaustive terms. In my writing I have used the term alternative medicine advisedly, agreeing with Saks that this term more accurately represents the 'socio-politically defined marginal standing (of therapies) in the healthcare system' (1991: 3). Where direct quotes have used these different terms I have left them unchanged. In-depth interviews took place throughout the North West of England with a total of thirty aromatherapists, reflexologists and osteopaths.

Alternative views of health

There has been an extensive debate over the last twenty to thirty years on the contested nature of the concept of health. Increasingly, health is conceptualised as complex, being multi-dimensional, multidisciplinary and holistic, and this understanding has been key to attempts to develop the role of public health (Baum 1998) and health promotion (Noack 1987) into the new millennium. Antonovsky (1993) argues for a model of health that incorporates an understanding of both the individual and social powers that shape health and disease. Embedded in this is a wide spectrum ranging from ease to disease, with ease suggesting a sense of coherence and belonging in the world and feeling supported. Holism is a central characteristic of alternative medicine (Fulder 1995), commonly recognised as the integration of the body-mind-spirit (Pietroni 1990) and has been influential in attempts to redefine health. However, the concept of vitalism, the vital force, or subtle energy fields, provokes a great deal of controversy within medicine. While used extensively in traditional systems of healing, in orthodox science they are both disputed and evasive to bio-medical science (Kaptchuk 1996). All these concepts are reflected when alternative practitioners are describing their work.

Holism

The majority of practitioners interviewed defined their practice as holistic. Susan talks about how the mind and body are integrated and how she deals with that in a reflexology treatment:

> if you get somebody and if they've got eczema, or psoriasis, there'll be reflexes that you'll work on for those areas, but also, if there's a background reason they've got eczema or psoriasis, say if it's stress related, if they can talk to you about their problems that they are having in work [for example], you can try and give them some pointers to either deal with their stresses, or if they can't eliminate them completely … perhaps approach their stresses in a different way. … that emotional thing can have a bearing on the physical. … It's just really making it holistic.

Rose sees a 'fit' between her aromatherapy training and her previous experience. This allows her to integrate and apply her knowledge:

> [training in aromatherapy] gives me a chance to bring in my degree in botany and biology and the bio-chemical side of that. My career since the early 1980s has been in the field of biological conservation, general ecology, [and] environmental education. … This has given me the chance to use the … knowledge about plants in a different way. And to combine it with the nursing experience I've had prior to that. I've always had an interest in … preventative healthcare and body awareness and to put those together in a way that, well, I find very fulfilling.

For the alternative practitioner a consultation involves an understanding of the lifestyle, behaviours and relationships of their clients. Colin describes what he is doing during an osteopathic consultation:

> So, it's looking at the body ... and the relationship of the parts to each other ... and you can do this through visual body reading ... patterns, distortions. You do it through movements, so what is moving freely, what's not, what's tight, what's restricted ... palpation, tissue tightnesses and muscle weaknesses and muscle imbalances. From that you can usually see where the patterns are coming from, postural strain, use of body, erm, trauma, stress, accident ... and you ask questions. A deeper layer is someone's lifestyle, occupation, relationships, money. ... Also people can be struggling with the meaning of life and that can be manifested in the body. That could be fear, rage, anger, jealousy ... either someone hasn't been licensed to express through, you know, childhood patterning, or it's unwise to express it, it's unsafe, or they haven't got the skills in expressing it, so it's got to be stuffed back down into the body, or it could be something out of consciousness where there's been experiences quite early on where it's been too painful. ... Long-term stress like responsibility, grinding people down, erm, any lack of emotional nurturance in someone's life. ... Trauma, to go back into trauma is just too frightening. ... I attract people who know how I work ... holistically.

For most osteopaths however, holism is more narrowly defined. A number of osteopaths alluded to the problem of how, with increasing professionalisation, the techniques that they use have, to some extent, become the focus of what they do. Yet a holistic approach was what attracted Sam into osteopathy:

> osteopathy is perceived as a technique, you know, we manipulate! Now the whole thing when I was training that got me interested and kept my enthusiasm going was the idea of looking at the body as a sort of interconnecting set of systems ... and again that was like holistic ... some of the people who influenced me the most when I was training did talk about a holistic way of looking at things. ... I don't think osteopaths are holistic because they are missing out on that, you know, emotional side of patients [which] is a major part of one's life. ... I mean osteopathy, when it talks about holistic ways of looking at things, just confines itself to the body, so if there's a knee pain we pat ourselves on the back because we happen to look at the neck. ... I think that's a very narrow version of holism.
>
> (Sam, osteopath)

Tom, however, was emphatic that osteopathy was denying its own history of vitalism:

> As a whole I think osteopathy is hiding it [its history] under the carpet, or is in denial about it in a way, because they did a lot of promotional stuff on modern physiology and all the rest of it to gain acceptance [by medicine]. ... at the end of the day, the difference between these complementary or alternative therapies and orthodox medicine is vitalism, that's the critical issue, and you can talk about holism till the cows come home but holism doesn't exist without vitalism. But the only limiting factor is your own personal belief system, so if you don't believe in the energetic model ... then your holistic view is only going to cover mechanical aspects [of osteopathy] and the mental aspect, including the emotional. Lots of people draw up their own model of holism ...

In interviews with practitioners, holism was found to be a central concept that is wholeheartedly embraced within aromatherapy and reflexology. For the osteopaths, however, it is a more difficult issue. While a number of the osteopaths claim holism as part of their work, increasing professionalisation has meant that some feel it is not part of their practice. Other osteopaths are frustrated with what they perceive as an attempt to subdue the concept to gain acceptance from allopathy.

Interconnectedness

Alternative medicine also draws on ideas from traditional systems of healing which recognise the interconnected nature of the individual within their environment. This may be expressed as an inner source, as below:

> I think it's two threads really. One is an interest in the natural world around, a great need to know more about the natural world and how it works, and that includes our bodies, and the other is a growing attachment to a, not a spiritual dimension, but an inner, an inner source we can tap into for healing and balance. And I think when those two come together you manage to do some good healing work, some good practitioner work ...
>
> (Rose, aromatherapist)

Or it can be expressed in a spiritual context. Pamela describes herself as a practising pagan and a 'non-form' (no particular religious base) witch. Her belief system provides the framework for the many therapies, herbalism, reflexology and various forms of healing practices, she incorporates into her practice:

> It is part of my tradition to use oils, plants and herbs ... and a witch is
> one who is able to work with forces of nature in order to bring about
> change ...

She works informally in her local community, clients are given treatment
for free or on an exchange of goods or skills basis. Pauline represents the
kind of practitioner who has a long history of alternative political, ideological, and now, spiritual traditions. When she first started training in
reflexology and aromatherapy she was a committed political and social
campaigner, having worked previously in the trade union movement, equal
opportunities and the political collective movement. Her involvement with
alternative therapies triggered an interest in alternative spiritualities also:

> coming from an alternative [background], ... [I'm] just a reactive type of
> person, I kind of kick up against things, so I was very much involved in
> Goddess spirituality ... Wicca, that was where I was coming from,
> promoting feminine spirituality. ... That's changed slightly ... but I'm
> still very much interested in the feminine aspect of spirituality but it's
> less ... I think I'm going more with the flow, the connectedness of every-
> thing.

> How do her beliefs affect her practice?

> It is connected. ... if people come for aromatherapy I don't talk unless
> they initiate a conversation but spiritual beliefs will often be part of the
> conversation. People come for reflexology [and] they're face to face. If
> they want to be quiet I'll be quiet but a lot of the time people will ask a
> question and we'll have this philosophical discussion, and I listen ... but
> it is an integral part, an important part of me. When we're having
> discussions as part of their therapeutic treatment that has to influence
> my responses ...

Richard makes explicit the link between the individual body and wider
systemic influences of health that are more implicit in the accounts above:

> ... some kind of systemic look at the body as a dynamic, you know,
> whole, where you're looking at the inter-relationship of the various parts
> and the pattern of stresses on the body in which physical manipulation
> forms one of the major forms of dealing with the body, and so it's a
> physically orientated intervention into a whole body dynamic system
> and it depends on how big you draw the system in which you place the
> body and allow social, emotional, environmental, political, and spiritual
> factors in.

For practitioners, alternative ideologies or spiritualities were important and identified as part of the personal legitimacy that they valued, and to be working holistically was part of that. The importance of spirituality was often emphasised, though that spirituality could take many forms and was used in almost free-form eclecticism, drawn from a diverse set of philosophies. So the practitioners allude to their practice as part of a wider alternative ideology, an active form of political and spiritual resistance against the excesses of consumer society, a way of simplifying their lives. This affiliation to diverse 'New Age' beliefs and practices, with its emphasis on self-defined spirituality, also has strong links with new social movements, such as the environmental and women's movements. Interestingly, a number of therapists also use the term 'green medicine', using these frameworks to provide a link to the message of green politics. Moving from a focus on the individual and their treatment, they are able to make links with the social and structural determinants of health. Scott (1996) noticed similarities between homeopathy and feminist agendas in their desire to integrate the personal, the political and the social. There are also broad similarities with the radical public health and health promotion movements (Braathen 1996). For example, Hancock's (1993) ecological model of health combines health, human development and the community ecosystem in a Mandala of Health. Here the determinants of health are presented as 'nested' with others, ranging from the biological and personal to the ecological and planetary, including the social and political. Labonte's (1991) concept of econology also has resonance here.

The promotion of health

Health promotion and the importance of preventative medicine was highly valued by the practitioners:

> it's more about how you can work with someone to promote health and what is involved in that process ... I think a lot of it [osteopathy] is about education and supporting people. And we do that in lots of different ways. ... Last week I had somebody whose sister has been diagnosed as diabetic and this patient was really worried and the backache had got worse recently. Now I'm not saying it's a cause and effect thing, that she's worried because her sister is a diabetic, but she was talking about it, she was bringing it into the room. ... so I talked to her. She didn't know much about diabetes, you know, ... so I was just chatting to her about that and gave her the number of the British Diabetic Association, there's a helpline and stuff. So, in a way, I think what we do as osteopaths is a bit like what GP's used to do, we'll sit down, spend time and educate people as to what symptoms mean.
>
> (John, osteopath)

Therapies were characterised as being preventative, working with the body to maintain a balance of health, a state of equilibrium. Hazel, was originally trained as a biomedical scientist but is now working as a part time reflexologist:

> [it is] important to look after your body as a whole, as in holistic therapies, not to just treat a symptom because you could be treating the symptom from here to eternity but you'd never get down to the root of the problem. So ... through the biomedical sciences you've got an understanding of the disease processes and ... how the system is going out of balance. But ... how does that system get out of balance in the first place? I think people are more aware of their own health and they have to take responsibility for themselves. ... It's the whole preventative therapy side. ... I think complementary therapy should be an on-going preventative thing.

Self healing and promoting the body's own healing mechanism was also alluded to, albeit expressed in a way that bio-medicine may not recognise:

> we've got channels of energy in our body ... and if these channels of energy are blocked, then you get ill and a blockage will show up as a pain in the foot, so by working on the painful areas we can clear those blockages and set your energy flowing again so it's really allowing self healing, promoting your body's own healing mechanism.
>
> (Gaye, reflexologist)

Multi-therapy practice

What was particularly noticeable about the aromatherapists and reflexologists was the wide range of therapies that they were trained in and which they used, usually interchangeably. This was facilitated by their adherence to vitalism as a core unitary principle underlying all their work. Thus the therapies were the vehicle by which they worked with the client at an energetic level. Vicky, for example, combines reflexology, baby massage, Indian head massage and Reiki: 'No therapy stands on its own but together they're stronger.'

I had defined Mary as an aromatherapist, prior to meeting her:

> Now, the way I've evolved ... I'm also a colour healer. I work with the chakras [energy centres] as well, and, you know, at some point during a treatment I always incorporate some colour with the energy centres, if not during the massage, then I always finish with it at the end, using colour, perhaps going through the colours of the rainbow with the energy centres, before I finish. It brings the energy from the colours into each energy centre, so there are certain colours that resonate energeti-

cally with each of the energy centres through the body and so it's another tool really … it's all part of the energetic clearing, the emotional clearing, clearing the blockages and encouraging strong energy flow.

In fact, I found that all the aromatherapists and the reflexologists were trained in a number of therapies. While, for the purposes of selecting therapists for my sample to interview, I had defined them as primarily one or the other, in reality there was a lot of crossover and increasingly I realised the problem of definition. The therapists often defined themselves in this way, largely, I felt, for legitimacy and convenience. I had selected Brenda as an aromatherapist to interview and found that she too struggled with this problem of definition:

I have struggled with it to be honest. I don't know what I am. I think I'm probably better categorised as a massage therapist who works with oils as well, though … at the Centre I work as an aromatherapist or as a massage therapist and I identify with the clients quite clearly, as I do here, what focus it is … and the clinical aspect obviously comes in, I suspect, when I've been trying to analyse what I do, it's not so much using the oils in an aromatherapy massage, I will do the massage I think is appropriate for that person and use oils to supplement that, but where it comes in clinically is providing oils and creams and advice in how to use oils in between treatments and that increasingly seems to be the way that I'm operating the aromatherapy.

While most of the osteopaths I interviewed clearly defined themselves as primarily osteopaths, Colin was different. He practises a whole range of different therapies and integrates them together. Trained in osteopathy, remedial massage, Reiki healing, psychotherapy, hypnotherapy, neuro-linguistic programming, and aspects of acupuncture and shiatsu, he explains the problem of defining himself, particularly to the osteopathic community:

I've trouble explaining that to people [that he integrates different therapies] so both colleagues, you know, who I trained with in osteopathy and other people, who have been in one discipline who, you know, 'I do acupuncture' or 'I do homeopathy, what do you do?', sort of, they struggle, and they either say, 'Oh it's too much, you can't do it', or 'Good luck', or kind of criticise me because of lack of boundaries … but I've said, well no, it's integrative, there is a pattern there, and … maybe you can't see it but I can. So now I'm quite [safe] being in this ground and I can defend it. So, for example, part of my training is understanding of the meridians, so, if I look at a body I can see where those lines [are], and

I can almost know what acupressure points are going to be the useful ones for me to use ... I don't use needles. I wouldn't call it shiatsu or acupressure but it's working with energy lines ... I like to have more than one way of treating people ... what's appropriate for that person.

In this account he is clearly describing how his work is underpinned by an energetic, or vitalistic, view of the body.

Empowerment

Empowerment is another strategy in health promotion that finds resonance within alternative medicine. WHO (1986) defined health promotion as: *'the process of enabling people to increase control over, and to improve their health'*. Debates have ensued in health promotion about the different meanings and levels of empowerment. Rappaport (1985) argues that empowerment does not occur when it is 'given' by the professional, but rather when it is taken by individuals and communities to enable them to set out and achieve their own agendas. In the interviews with alternative practitioners it was clear that they felt, first, a sense of personal empowerment through the training and work that they did; and, second, that they were able to contribute their skills in a number of different work settings, many of which were in local, community-based projects. However, such work tended to be informal and ad hoc in nature.

Personal empowerment

The history of the professionalisation of healing is linked to the relegation of women to the role of healthcare provider (Achterberg 1990; Brooke 1993), and this is predominantly seen as a gender struggle (Chamberlain 1981). The practice of aromatherapy and reflexology can also be regarded as highly gendered and investigation of this division of labour is an aspect of the research being undertaken. Interviews with alternative practitioners found that alternative medicine, as a career, was attractive because there appeared to be flexible and creative modes of working that were particularly, though not exclusively, suited to women's skills. Motivations for practising alternative medicine were diverse, but included flexible working practices; the desire to work with people and help others; espousal of an alternative work ethic; personal development and dislike of working in large bureaucratic organisations. The ability to be self-employed, as well as using entrepreneurial skills also seemed to be a great attraction.

All the practitioners interviewed were self-employed. Hazel, when I interviewed her, was on maternity leave from her NHS post:

one of the reasons why I decided to take up the course, reflexology, because that was, I wanted something that was going to be more flexible, ... and to be able to keep up my actual job as a biomedical scientist as a part-time role, because I get the stability there, a regular salary and to keep my experience in there as well. ... [but the] problem with the NHS, is the fact that you don't see any prospects, you know, for promotion ... although in the end I decided ... I didn't really just want a career, as in to further myself in that way. I wanted to further myself in a more personal way. Something that I valued more, that I could get satisfaction out of ...

Hazel's intention is to build up her private practice to a point where she can leave her NHS job; this was a feature of many of the interviews. Training in therapies was part of a strategy towards building a business and leaving their 'day job'. Rose saw training in both aromatherapy and reflexology as a way to redirect her workpath:

I think from the beginning I wanted to get to where I was able to put the work I was doing behind me. ... And all the time I was doing my training and starting to work a bit with private clients in the evening and so on and it had this kind of tunnel effect whereby I realised I'm going to be able to widen out and do my own thing instead and be much more grounded and get away from the situation. And I did ...

For Brenda, a senior teacher and education inspector for many years, aromatherapy training afforded a complete shift in her thinking:

I suppose it just released so much that was pent up inside me – I came from a non-touch family – and to have that was a Eureka moment ... there was a bit of me that was aware I didn't want to do what I was doing for ever ... and this seemed a lovely way of getting out of the academic and just switching from this managerial, academic focus into something which had its own challenges but was completely different. A completely different mode. I wasn't considering, when I did the training, where it would take me. It was once I hit 50, and enhanced pensions were still around then, both my children had just finished university, my husband was in Birmingham, and it seemed to be a watershed. I was having to apply for my own job, yet again ... and I was also spending more and more time pushing paper and going to meetings and then being involved with policy, ... whereas really I wanted to be involved with people ... that was one of the major things ...

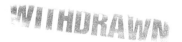

This theme of working with people was important to all the therapists:

> 'I have no idea where osteopathy came from ... the idea of self-employment seemed like a good one ... [and] I liked the idea of working with bodies and people.
>
> (John, osteopath).

Therapists expressed feelings of being in control and freedom that self-employment brought:

> I went fully independent. I was so excited about it, I saw it as a freedom. For the first time there was going to be only me to tell me what to do, only me to report to ... it was quite scary but quite exciting at the same time and I planned for it. I didn't go into it not knowing what to do ... I can take control a lot more effectively of my life ...
>
> (Rose, reflexologist)

Pauline has extensive caring responsibilities but runs her own private practice and nationally accredited training school in aromatherapy:

> I do something I enjoy and most people don't have that do they? I love it. I love it. I love the people, I like the people who come to me ... I can pick and choose when I want to work, when I don't want to work, within limits ... and I earn enough to pay the bills ... but I'm established now, I'm lucky.

Mary, a single parent, represents the entrepreneurial spirit among many therapists. In the past she has run a number of small, successful business ventures in the local area and now runs a growing alternative therapies practice in a small village:

> I've been finding out what works and what doesn't in terms of advertising and getting known. I've put a tremendous amount of energy into it in the last twelve months ... for about two months during the summer, every weekend I was somewhere doing a stall, promoting the Centre. ... I don't think I was realistic about how long it took to build up so in order to do this I had to have a big mortgage. ... I'm optimistic that with the combined rents of the therapists, and my own practice of massage, I think I will cover all my overheads by September the way things are going, which is nearly a year since opening ...

Many therapists, however, expressed difficulties with dealing with the financial aspects of their practices. In contrast to Mary, another practitioner, Sophie, who had also set up a private clinic, in a city, was finding the market difficult. Little research has, as yet, been carried on this aspect of alternative medicine.

Working toward community empowerment?

An interesting aspect of the research was that practitioners were engaged in a mixed economy of work. Predominantly, their practices were based in the private sector and some osteopaths carried out a small amount of NHS work, although this was seen as quite problematic. My focus here, however, is on the significant number of practitioners working in the voluntary, non-statutory sectors. Gaye, a reflexologist works with a range of groups in the community:

> That's why my, er, practice has developed in the way that it has because I found at the beginning that the people who most need it can't afford it. So I introduced concessions for the elderly and the unemployed ... a social worker that was on the [name] Community Health Project saw my advert and was organising an event for [area of a city] and she phoned me up and said would you like to come to this Asian Women's afternoon? And that led to so many different events. ... working with the Asian women went on for a few years, the money's run out now ... the Project is coming to a close ... people would come in and we were paid for going but they got their therapy for free, just to see what it was like. ... I actually work as a regular at [a women's centre], I do there every Thursday morning and the [name] Centre every Wednesday morning, and the people there, if they are unemployed get half-price treatments.

Brenda's work also has a strong focus on working with groups in the community. Two days a week are spent working as a therapist in a local Mental Health Centre, partly funded through the local Health Action Zone (HAZ). The local therapists got together and set up an association of complementary therapies in the local region for mutual support and to make themselves more visible. This strategy seemed to be successful:

> A lot of organisations are beginning to approach us and ask us to do talks. There's a whole range of people involved, reflexology, aromatherapy massage, Reiki, crystal healing, hypnotherapy, homeopathy, shiatsu ... and we've had a grant through working with different organisations. We've been able to offer some therapies to [the] elderly Asian population in the [name] Centre and also to a charity that was set up to support people with children with disabilities ... and then going in and working with a youth group and just providing a bit of foot massage here and there to introduce them to it ... there's so much community funding, we're in the process of trying to get involved with the ... SRB [Social Regeneration Budget] but there is also a health initiative because this area is one of the focused areas.

Therapists viewed money from initiatives such as HAZ's and the SRB as a way of supporting their private practice, while also working in community settings. Such work, however, appeared to be uncoordinated and rather informal at times, and often it was on a voluntary, unpaid basis. Colin articulates some working models for provision of alternative medicine in communities:

'HB's [name] drop-in centres are non-expert-driven where people gradually come and start being aware of different ways of working with themselves ... LG's [name] work [is] community therapeutics where it's training people [in] basic skills, you know, physical skills around therapy massage, listening skills, counselling and exercise, and they can be quite useful people in the community ... there's money coming through different kinds of centres, Healthy Living Centres, Health Action Zones. You know this kind of private sector initiative might just take off. ... Obviously the NHS holds the purse strings but I think to wait for them is not the answer ...

Colin felt that it was for practitioners to organise themselves and become pro-active in community work. What appeared to be a problem for the formal bodies was the issue of contract conditions and pay, as well as visibility of, and access to, practitioners. Colin is active in his region in building links and lobbying for conditions for practitioners employed in the statutory and non-statutory sectors:

There's lots of pitfalls at the moment in that PCG's [primary care groups] don't know how to contract therapists, what we are trying to do ... is to get contracts on the agenda.

Local authority reorganisation of services, and HAZ agendas of social inclusion, equity and innovation, increasingly are informed through a social model of health which has clear parallels with the work that alternative practitioners are already engaging in. From the practitioners' perspective, what was clear was that they saw these initiatives as a mechanism for working inclusively with a wide range of disadvantaged groups. How far this commitment is being recognised within the statutory sector has yet to be explored, alongside investigation into partnership working and how effectively, or otherwise, as Colin suggests, this is being done.

Conclusion

Through accounts drawn from alternative practitioners, it is clear that quite a large amount of their work involves promoting health with both individuals and individuals within their community contexts. Despite the fact that the majority of alternative healthcare is practised, and consumed, in the private sector, what these interviews have also demonstrated is an awareness that alternative medicine has a potential to provide a bridge between individual treatment and social medicine, both ideologically and in practice. The voluntary and non-statutory sectors in health promotion do seem to increasingly recognise the value that alternative medicine has, and are harnessing the enthusiasm and energy of its practitioners. Healthy public policy initiatives, such as Healthy Living Centres, Sure Start and New Deal for Communities, are also recognising this potential. The challenge, and danger, for the future is to harness this creativity in a way that values the core tenets of holism and vitalism in alternative medicine, and nurtures the work that alternative practitioners do, rather than exploiting it. For both sets of practitioners to develop a shared vision for working together requires a shift in culture for health services and health providers, both ideologically and in work practices. Debates about integration of alternative medicine have largely been led by the medical lobby and are focused on incorporation or assimilation into the NHS. In this way, the biomedical paradigm stays intact. If, however, we locate the practice of alternative medicine within a salutogenic, health-promoting paradigm, this immediately changes the tenor of the debate. From this perspective, we can harness the 'on the ground' demand for therapies and provide a system of health and well-being that is participatory, collaborative and health-promoting. It also changes the research questions with which we might engage. Alternative medicine has the potential to strengthen and enhance the work that health promoters are attempting in communities, while health promoters can recognise that there is a ready-made network of community-based, health-promoting practitioners. This can only enhance a radical public health agenda.

References

Achterberg, J. (1990) *Woman as Healer*. Boston, MA: Shambhala.

Antonovsky, A. (1993) 'The Sense of Coherence as a Determinant of Health', in A. Beattie (ed.) *Health and Wellbeing: A Reader*. Milton Keynes: Open University Press.

Bakx, K. (1991) 'The Eclipse of Folk Medicine in Western Society', *Sociology of Health and Illness* 13(1): 20–38.

Baum, F. (1998) *The New Public Health: An Australian Perspective*. South Melbourne, Australia: Oxford University Press.

Benor, D. (1995) 'Spiritual Healing: A Unifying Influence in Complementary Therapies', *Complementary Therapies in Medicine* 3: 234–8.

Braathen, E. (1996) 'Communicating the Individual and the Body Politic: The Discourse on Disease Prevention and Health Promotion in Alternative Therapies', in S. Cant and U. Sharma (eds.) *Complementary and Alternative Medicines: Knowledge in Practice*, London: FAB Press, pp. 151–62.

Brooke, E. (1993) *Women Healers through History*. London: The Women's Press.

Bryden, H. (ed.) (1999) 'A Participant's Synopsis of Human Healing: Perspectives, Alternatives and Controversies', unpublished, available at www.adhom.org.

Chamberlain, M. (1981) *Old Wives' Tales: Their History, Remedies and Spells.* London: Virago.

Coward, R. (1989) *The Whole Truth: The Myth of Alternative Health.* London: Faber.

Department of Health (DoH) (1999) *Making a Difference.* London: DoH.

Dickenson, D.P. (1996) 'The Growth of Complementary Therapy: A Consumer-Led Boom', in E. Ernst (ed.) *Complementary Medicine: An Objective Appraisal.* Oxford and Boston, MA: Butterworth-Heinemann, pp. 150–61.

Donnelly, D. (2001) 'Read My Lips: Integration, Integration, Integration, the Seamless Web of Joined-Up Thinking', unpublished paper presented to the Alternative and Complementary Healthcare Research Network (ACHRN) Seminar Series, 18 May 2001, Salford University, UK.

Emslie, M., Campbell, M. and Walkes, K. (1996) 'Complementary Therapies in a Local Healthcare Setting, Part 1: Is There a Real Public Demand, *Complementary Therapies in Medicine* 4(1): 39–42.

Ernst, E. (1996) *Complementary Medicine: An Objective Appraisal.* Oxford and Boston, MA: Butterworth-Heinemann.

Ernst, E. and White, A. (2000) 'The BBC Survey of Complementary Medicine Use in the UK', *Complementary Therapies in Medicine* 8: 32–6.

Foundation for Integrated Medicine (FIM) (2002) 'Regulation Series Seminars', *Integrated Health* 10(April).

Fulder, S. (1995) The Impact of Alternative Medicine on Our Views of Health', *Journal of Contemporary Health* winter: 24 vol. 1.

Fulder, S. (1996) *The Handbook of Alternative and Complementary Medicine.* London: Oxford University Press.

Furnham, A. and Bhagrath, R. (1993) 'A Comparison of Health Beliefs and Behaviours of Clients of Orthodox and Complementary Medicine', *British Journal of Clinical Psychology* 32: 237–46.

Goldstein, M.S. (2000) 'The Culture of Fitness and the Growth of CAM', in M. Kelner *et al.* (eds) *Complementary and Alternative Medicine: Challenge and Change.* Amsterdam: Harwood Academic Press.

Hancock, T. (1993) 'Health, Human Development and the Community Eco-System: Three Ecological Models,' *Health Promotion International* 8(1): 41–7.

House of Lords Select Committee on Science and Technology (2000) *Sixth Report: Complementary and Alternative Medicine.* London: HMSO.

Kelner, M. and Wellman, B. (1997) 'Health Care and Consumer Choice: Medical and Alternative Therapies', *Social Science and Medicine* 45(2): 203–12.

Kaptchuk, T.J. (1996) 'Historical Context of the Concept of Vitalism in Complementary and Alternative Medicine', in M. Micozzi (ed.) *Fundamentals of Complementary and Alternative Medicine.* pp 35–48.

Labonte, R. (1991) 'Econology: Integrating Health and Sustainable Development, Part 1: Theory and Background', *Health Promotion International* pp 35-48 6(1): 49–65.

Mills, S. and Budd, S. (2000) 'Professional Organisation of Complementary and Alternative Medicine in the United Kingdom', A Second Report to the Department of Health, University of Exeter.

Mills, S. and Peacock, W. (1997) 'Professional organisations of Complementary and Alternative Medicine in the United Kingdom', The Centre for Complementary Health Studies, Exeter University, UK.

MORI (1989) 'Research on Alternative Medicine', conducted for *The Times*.

Morris, S. (1996) ' "A Very Privileged Position": Metaphors Used by Complementary Therapists Receiving NHS Oncology Referrals', *Journal of Contemporary Health* 4 (summer): 53–5.

NHS Confederation (1997) 'Complementary Medicine in the NHS: Managing the Issues', *Research Paper No. 4*. London: NHS Confederation.

Noack, H. (1987) 'Concepts of Health and Health Promotion', in T. Abelin, Z. Brzezinski and V. Carstairs (eds) *Measurement in Health Promotion and Protection*, WHO Regional Publications, European Series No. 22. Copenhagen: WHO.

Owen, D.K., Lewith, G., Stephens, C.R. (2001) 'Can Doctors Respond to Patients' Increasing Interest in Complementary and Alternative Medicine?', *British Medical Journal* 322: 154–8.

Pietroni, P. (1990) *The Greening of Medicine*. London: Gollancz.

Raeburn, J. and Rootman, I. (1998) *People-Centred Health Promotion*. London: Wiley.

Rappaport, J. (1985) 'The Power of Empowerment Language', *Social Policy* 16: 15–21.

Royal London Homeopathic Hospital (1999) *The Evidence Base of Complementary Medicine*, 2nd edn. London: Royal London Homeopathic Hospital.

Saks, M. (ed.) (1991) *Alternative Medicine in Britain* . London: Clarendon Press.

Saks, M. (2000) 'Professionalisation, Politics and CAM', in M. Kelner *et al.* (eds) *Complementary and Alternative Medicine: Challenge and Change*. Amsterdam: Harwood Academic Press.

Scheid, V. (1993) 'Orientalism Revisited: Reflections on Scholarship, Research and Professionalisation', *European Journal of Oriental Medicine* 1(2): 23–33.

Scott, A. (1996) 'Body Politics: Homeopathy as a Feminist Form of Medicine', paper presented at the Social Aspects of Complementary Medicine Conference, Derby University, April.

Scrambler, G. (2002) *Health and Social Change: A Critical Theory*. Milton Keynes: Open University Press.

Sharma, U. (1995) *Complementary Medicine Today: Practitioner and Patients*. London: Routledge.

Springett, J. (2001) 'Appropriate Approaches to the Evaluation of Health Promotion', *Critical Public Health* 11(2) 139–51.

Stone, J. (2001) 'How Might Traditional Remedies be Incorporated into Discussions of Integrated Medicine?', *Complementary Therapies in Nursing and Midwifery* 7(2): 55–8.

Stone, J. and Matthews, J. (1995) 'The Effective Regulation of Complementary Medicine', *Complementary Therapies in Medicine* 3: 175–8.

Stone, J. and Matthews, J. (1996) *Complementary Medicine and the Law*. Oxford: Oxford University Press.

Vickers, A. *et al.* (1997) quoted in A.F. Long and G. Mercer 'Challenges in Researching the Effectiveness of Complementary Therapies', *Journal of Contemporary Health* 8(winter 2000): 13–19.

Vincent, C., Furnham, A. and Willsmore, M. (1995) 'The Perceived Efficacy of Complementary and Orthodox Medicine in Complementary and General Practice Patients', *Health Education Research* 10(4): 395–405.

WHO (1986) *The Ottawa Charter for Health Promotion*. Geneva: WHO.

Chapter 11

The growing social significance of health promotion in twentieth-century Scotland

David Player and Peter Murray

The first half of the twentieth century

> By 1900, after a protracted struggle, Scotland had come to accept the need for publicly run and funded systems of public health surveillance, drainage, water supply and medical care both for paupers and for those suffering from certain highly infectious diseases. ... In retrospect it seems reasonably clear that what was at stake in the nineteenth century was the survival of modern industrial, urban civilization in this country.
>
> (Brotherston 1987)

So wrote Sir John Brotherston, Chief Medical Officer for Scotland in his introduction to *Improving the Common Weal: Aspects of Scottish Health Services 1900–1984*.

In fact the twentieth century was ushered in by a stark reminder of just how much was at stake. The Boer War (1899–1902) cruelly exposed the poor state of health of British and especially Scottish troops. During recruitment for the Boer War in Scotland almost 50 per cent of recruits from poor backgrounds were declared unfit on physical grounds. It was typical of the period that this was seen principally as a threat to the 'defence of the realm'.

However it could be argued that the conservatism of the age was compounded by Scotland's constitutional position within the United Kingdom. As Brotherston argues in *Improving the Common Weal*:

> Since 1707 all Scottish legislation had had to pass through a Parliament largely composed of men who knew little of Scotland. The natural consequence of this was that much needed reforms were often considerably delayed .... The parliamentary union ... did not encourage the adoption of distinctively Scottish solutions to new problems.... The in-built conservatism of this constitutional arrangement naturally suited conservative interests in Scotland.
>
> (1987: 5–6)

It could be argued that this tendency persisted to various degrees throughout the twentieth century, being modified at various times when there was a UK-wide movement for reform, such as after the great Labour landslide of 1945. At the end of the twentieth century, the creation of the Scottish Parliament held the promise of providing a Scottish response not merely to 'new problems' but to the familiar Scottish scourges of poverty and poor health.

Nevertheless, in the early years of the twentieth century, radicals such as Drs McVail, Mackenzie and Alison, were pushing against conservative interests and advocating in favour of the poor and their health. They pressed for a review of the Poor Laws and medical relief for the poor. Even at this time, however, the Labour Party had abandoned the idea of a special medical service for the poor and were looking at the concept of a comprehensive medical service for all. But it was the more conservatively minded Scots and Britons who were becoming concerned and worried about the growing numbers of the poor and the increasing costs of supporting them.

Thus it was a Tory, not a Liberal government, which appointed a Royal Commission in 1905 to look at the Poor Law and recommend necessary reforms. The Scottish report of the Royal Commission was presented in 1909. While it was acknowledged that reform was desirable, the majority were not in favour of radical changes. Although they recommended abolition of parish councils and the transference of Poor Law medical relief to county and large burgh councils, they maintained that Poor Law medical relief should deal only with paupers. The minority report, though, supported by Fabians such as Beatrice Webb, recommended the public health and preventative approach to medical care which would cover all classes in the community. Interestingly, this latter approach was also supported by all the distinguished public health officials of the day, including Dr Leslie Mackenzie, medical member of the Local Government Board for Scotland and Dr John McVail, the Royal Commission's own medical investigator. The minority report was vigorously attacked in *Glasgow Herald*, which said that it 'embodies a wholly impractical socialism' and voiced concern about 'the effects on the national character of this elaborate process of wholesale relief' (2 Nov. 1909). The public health approach allied to local government reform of the Poor Laws was thus delayed for another twenty years.

The pusillanimity shown by the Commission annoyed the Chancellor of the Exchequer, David Lloyd George, who was convinced that the key to improving healthcare lay in a state-supported health insurance scheme. The result of his efforts was the National Insurance Act of 1911. The application of this Act in Scotland was supervised by the Scottish Insurance Commission. The Act covered unemployment as well as health insurance, provided medical benefit to all insured persons and voluntary contributors earning less than £160 per annum (Mackintosh 1953).

Before the outbreak of war in August 1914 there were two other relevant pieces of Scottish legislation. The first was the Highlands and Islands (Medical

Services) Act of 1913. These sparsely populated areas, where many of the inhabitants lived barely above subsistence level, had been poorly served with medical, nursing and financial help. As a result of the Act, the Treasury granted a sum of £42,000 to induce enough doctors to practise in the crofting counties on the condition that the doctors agreed to attend, at reduced fees, patients belonging to the crofter class, their dependants and those of similar economic standing. The scheme was a success and the Highlands and Islands Medical Service was cherished by the Scottish Board of Health and its successor, the Department of Health for Scotland. This success played a significant part in the relatively cordial relationships between doctors in Scotland and the Department of Health for Scotland in the run-up to the National Health Service (Scotland) Act 1947, when compared with those between doctors in England and their Department of Health in London. The second piece of legislation was the Education (Scotland) Act of 1913 which established the School Medical Service.

The First World War saw three further Acts in Scotland. The Notification of Births (Extension) Act of 1915 made the notification of all births compulsory and empowered local authorities to attend to the health of expectant mothers, nursing mothers and children under five. The Midwives (Scotland) Act of 1915, provided for the much-needed registration of midwives, and the establishment of a Central Midwives Board for Scotland with wide powers for the training and control of midwives (no more Sarah Gamps). The Maternity and Child Welfare Act of 1918 empowered local authorities to provide hospitals for the care of expectant mothers and children under five.

The condition of housing in Scotland was recognised, at long last, in the *Report of the Royal Commission on the Housing of the Industrial Population of Scotland, Rural and Urban* in 1917. The relationship between poor health, bad housing and poverty is irrefutable. The one-roomed house had twice the infant mortality rate and three times the death rate from tuberculosis as the four-roomed house.

In practice the Housing (Scotland) Act of 1919 provided local authorities with a state subsidy for the building of council houses. By 1923, only 25,000 houses had been built. The Housing (Scotland) Act of 1924 increased the total subsidy. It was mainly the work of John Wheatley, Labour MP for Shettleston, and Minister of Health and Housing in the first Labour government. It stimulated an increase of 140 per cent over the number of houses built over the previous five-year period. By 1939 and the outbreak of the Second World War, almost 337,000 houses had been built, of which two-thirds were council houses, but this was still insufficient. Compared with housing in England, Scotland has always lagged far behind. In 1911, 8 per cent of the population of England lived in one- and two- roomed houses; in Scotland the figure was 50 per cent. By 1935, 22 per cent of Scottish houses were overcrowded while in some Clyde Valley towns the figure reached 40 per cent. In England, on the other hand, the national average figure was 3.8 per cent and the worst figure, in Sunderland, was 20.6 per cent. By 1936 there were still 300,000 houses in Scotland without modern sanitary conveniences (Parliamentary Debates 1905).

During the inter-war years, the numbers of people in Scotland living in poverty increased. The proportion unemployed in Scotland quickly overtook that in England, as did the proportion of those on Poor Law relief. There was a slowing down of the decrease in infant mortality rates when compared with England. There was a change in the composition of welfare rolls. Before 1914 few areas had more than 5 per cent of their population on these rolls, and some of the highest percentages could be found in the Highlands and Islands. After 1920, rolls grew remarkably. In some districts of Glasgow, such as Cowcaddens, Gorbals and Bridgeton, the Poor Law disabled roll accounted for 40 per cent of the population (Brown and Cook 1983).

Eventually, by the 1930s, general anxiety about Scotland's health problems and poverty was accentuated by general health statistics for Scotland, which compared unfavourably with England and other European countries (*Glasgow Herald* 6 April 1936).

It was into this atmosphere that the eagerly awaited *Report of the Committee on Scottish Health Services* was introduced on 1 July 1936 (known as the Cathcart Report, after its chairman Professor Cathcart of Glasgow University). Its main theme was the need for a national health policy. It advocated comprehensive changes in health education and promotion, increased provision for physical recreation and training, improvement in poor Scottish diet, revision of public health legislation to combat environmental hazards and improve sanitary standards, and pointed to the significance of the ageing population in terms of health service provision (Department of Health for Scotland 1936).

The Cathcart Report also endorsed the idea that the family doctor/general practitioner should be the focus of the health service and that local authority services should be given the task of co-ordination. It judged that the National Health Insurance scheme had been a success, that a separate domiciliary medical service for the poor was undesirable and that local authorities should be empowered to provide medical help for the 'necessitous'. Further, these arrangements should: 'ensure that as far as possible, poverty will not interrupt continuity of medical supervision by the family doctor' (Department of Health for Scotland 1936: 219–21).

Political reaction was less than enthusiastic. Thus Sir John Brotherston, Scotland's Chief Medical Officer, could write: 'the main obstacle to progress was not economic depression but absence of political will. This will was to be created by the experiences of the nation during Hitler's war' (McLachlan 1987).

The impact of the Second World War

With the passing of the Civil Defence Act of 1939, the Department of Health for Scotland took an active part in the supervision of the medical work of local authorities, emergency services, hospital and domiciliary, and evacuation of children and their mothers from vulnerable and crowded industrial areas. The evacuation at the beginning of the war, and again in 1941 after the air-raids on Clydeside, proved a shock, not just to those evacuated but to those areas receiving them and the workers organising it. Among children registered for evacuation from Glasgow, 30 per cent of clothing was bad or deplorable, 31 per cent were found to be infested with vermin, scabies, impetigo and the like. Some 5–10 per cent of evacuated children were enuretic and dirty habits involving a failure to use elementary sanitary and toilet facilities were wide-spread. Scabies was effectively dealt with by Medical Officers of Health using the Scabies Order (Scotland) of 1941 and low levels of immunisation against diphtheria were tackled with vigour. War produced the required resolution which had been absent in peacetime. By June 1942, 792,000 school children and pre-school children had been immunised against diphtheria, which represented 73 per cent of school children and 58 per cent of pre-school children. This represented a very substantial increase in take-up and, as a result, cases of diphtheria fell from 15,069 in 1946 to 5,679 in 1955 (MacNalty 1955).

The picture was different with pulmonary tuberculosis; the number of cases rose quite dramatically during the course of the war, reaching a peak of 7,316 cases in 1945 and extra beds had to be provided. As a result, mass radiography was introduced in Glasgow and Lanarkshire in 1944 allowing for early diagnosis and treatment.

Nutrition was to prove of extreme importance during the war and the work of Sir John Boyd Orr of Aberdeen was crucial. In his book *Food, Health and Income* he found that, although the Scottish diet had improved markedly since before the First World War, the diet of nearly half the population, while sufficient to satisfy hunger, was deficient for the maintenance of health (McNalty 1955: 234).

As a result of his investigations, food and rationing policies were framed to promote a balanced diet and *equal access to essential foods irrespective of income level*. The Scientific Advisory Committee of the Secretary of State for Scotland found improved levels of national health from 1941 onwards, and also found that: 'compared with pre-war diet, the food of workers – as well as their families – had improved' (McNalty 1955: 275).

For example, the consumption of milk increased by 45 per cent during the war due to the 'Milk in Schools Scheme'. By the end of the war, 68 per cent of Scottish children attending education authority schools were receiving free milk and 75 per cent of pregnant mothers, nursing mothers and pre-school children were participating in the National Milk Scheme. (McNalty 1955: 278). Together with the much improved provision of free school meals under the Education (Scotland) Act of 1942, such measures had a very significant effect on the health of infants and children during the war. There was a measurable improvement throughout the war in the heights and weights of children on entering and leaving school, and the improvement in health and expectation of life of infants and pre-school children between 1941 and 1946 was remarkable. For example, the infant mortality rate declined by 35 per cent between 1941 and 1946 – the greatest reduction since records were first kept in 1855 (McNalty 1955: 307).

In anticipation of high civilian and military casualties, the Emergency Medical Service (EMS) was set up, resulting in the provision of an extra 20,000 beds (approximately a 60 per cent increase in numbers) either in new hospitals or in additions to existing ones. There was a similar increase in back-up specialist services, in addition to the setting up of the Scottish National Blood Transfusion Service in 1940 and an Emergency Pathological Laboratory Service. Fortunately, the expected number of military and civilian casualties did not occur and the Secretary of State for Scotland, Tom Johnston, instructed that these increased services should be made freely available to all categories of war-workers who could not afford specialist diagnosis and treatment. By the middle of 1945, 32,826 patients had been taken off voluntary hospital waiting lists and treated in Emergency Medical Service hospitals (Department of Health for Scotland 1944).

It became clear to Tom Johnston and the Department of Health for Scotland that:

> The manpower needs of the nation required the organisation of the civilian medical service on lines which would secure that early and correct diagnosis and treatment were available for any condition which threatened to impair the working capacity of war-workers or leave a war aftermath of chronic invalidism.
>
> (Department of Health for Scotland 1944: 69)

To promote the implementation of this concept, Tom Johnston launched the Clyde Basin experiment in January 1942, and made it Scotland-wide in December 1942 under what was to be known as the Supplementary Medical Service Scheme. It is fair to say, therefore, that the foundations of the NHS in Scotland were well and truly laid during the war.

The National Health Service

The momentous publication of the Beveridge Report on Social Insurance and Allied Services on 1 December 1942 transformed thinking on poverty and health. Beveridge talked about five giants that had to be slain. These were: Want, Disease, Ignorance, Squalor and Idleness. The Report proposed a single unified social security scheme which would insure against interruption of earning power, whether because of sickness, disability, old age, unemployment or injury. In return for flat-rate contributions, benefits would be paid 'guaranteeing the minimum income needed for subsistence' (Beveridge 1942).

The whole structure rested upon three assumptions, the second of which, Assumption B, stated that a comprehensive health service would be made available to all. There was a three-day debate in the House of Commons on the Beveridge Report in February 1943. While the government refused to be stampeded into accepting all the recommendations, they did accept the commitment to a reorganised and comprehensive health service. The government at the time preferred a service mainly based on local authority control, but the British Medical Association were opposed to this idea and preferred a system of *ad hoc* authorities and central control.

As far as primary care was concerned, the government wanted a system based on health centres and a full-time salaried service. In Scotland, the Secretary of State Tom Johnston, was anxious to accommodate the general practitioners and urged concessions on the points of local authority control and a salaried service, anticipating the compromises to be made by Aneurin Bevan, the Minister of Health in the post-war Labour government. Political expediency in the end determined that Bevan and Joseph Westwood, the then Secretary of State for Scotland, would support a National Health Service (NHS) which had jettisoned local authority control for central control, and in which general practitioners were to be self-employed rather than part of a salaried service. The National Health Service (Scotland) Act 1947 and the National Health Service Act 1946 (for England and Wales) would come into effect on 5 July 1948 and were in most essentials the same.

The NHS offered the people of Britain a comprehensive medical service provided free, in the sense that patients did not have to pay for services, medicines or other aids at the time they were given them. The new service was warmly welcomed in Scotland and throughout Britain, with the British people, according to the *Glasgow Herald*: 'taking a pride in leading the world in progressive citizenship and in demonstrating what unregimented democracy could achieve' (5 July 1948).

As expected there was a rush to benefit from the new service at first. Doctors' surgeries were overcrowded; in the first year of the NHS, the number of prescriptions issued had increased threefold to 15 million and the average cost of prescriptions was 50 per cent higher than in the last year of the old National Health Insurance Scheme. The demand for dental services was very heavy and the cost had greatly exceeded expectations. Similarly, the demand for ophthalmic services was 'overwhelming', being five or six times what was estimated before Parliament approved the National Health Service Act.

Aneurin Bevan showed no remorse whatsoever, indeed he wrote:

> The new health service is a triumphant example of the superiority of collective action and public initiative applied to a segment of society (the sick) where commercial principles are seen at their worst. ... the free health service therefore represented pure socialism.
>
> (Bevan 1948)

Bevan was also the Minister for Housing and the same twin portfolio was held in Scotland. It was in this context that many of Scotland's public health specialists drew attention, at the end of the 1940s, to the great number of Scots living in 'single ends' (a dwelling situated within a tenement block, which comprised just one room for a whole family to eat and sleep in, and which lacked bathroom and toilet facilities, a communal WC was shared among many families) and declared that a healthy, decent life was no more possible under such conditions than in the nineteenth century. In essence, a medical service in such conditions was a form of 'elastoplast medicine' when what was needed was environmental and social improvement. This was aptly summed up by Professor T. Ferguson of the Department of Public Health at Glasgow University: 'To pour social and medical services into those wretched places was certainly uneconomic and often quite useless. Bad housing was still the greatest blot on Scotland's social welfare' (*The Scotsman* 6 Oct. 1949). Even by 1967, a third of Scottish families were still living in inadequate accommodation. The 1971 census showed that Scotland had 77.5 per cent of Britain's worst 5 per cent of socially deprived areas (Harvie 1981).

Apart from the NHS the other two assumptions on which the Beveridge Report was based were the provision of universal social security and family allowances, and the maintenance of a high level of employment. The concept of social security meant the guarantee by government to all its citizens of an income sufficient to ensure an agreed minimum standard of living. To attain this there were three underlying principles: universalism, comprehensiveness and adequacy. As we shall see, Beveridge's 'brave new world' faltered, and some would say failed, for a number of reasons, including a failure to maintain full employment, economic storms in Britain (and the world) and growing awareness of the inconsistencies regarding the principles of universalism and adequacy. In the latter case, Beveridge compromised with the Treasury regarding subsistence levels. He admitted that any estimate of subsistence income could not be scientific and had to be to some extent a matter of judgement. In the event he settled for flat-rate benefits which were in fact lower than Rowntree's levels for absolute poverty:

> With the passage of time, the Beveridge Report was indeed to be exposed as a flawed blueprint for the eradication of poverty. ... The major practical limitation was the attempt to base an extremely expensive system of relief (universal benefits) on a very restricted source of income (flat-rate contributions tied to what the poorest worker could afford).There was also the assumption of full employment.
>
> (Lowe 1993)

'Rediscovery' of poverty in 1965: the concept of relative poverty and the health divide

During the 1950s, there was growing concern within government, and among academics and some left-wing politicians, that the social security system was failing the poor. The most significant event in the debate was the publication on Christmas Eve 1965 of *The Poor and the Poorest* by Peter Townsend and Brian Abel-Smith, in which they claimed that the number living in poverty, far from decreasing under the welfare state, had increased from a minimum of 600,000 in 1953–4 to 2 million in 1964. The concept of poverty which they used, that of relative poverty, was not original to them; indeed it was the supposed guru of the right-wing think-tank, the Adam Smith Institute, who wrote in his *The Wealth of Nations* in 1812:

> By necessities I understand not just commodities which are indispensably necessary for the support of life, but whatever the custom of a country renders it indecent for creditable people, even of the lowest order, to be without.
>
> (Smith 1812)

Thus, in the Scotland of his day, Adam Smith included as necessities such items as a pair of leather shoes and two linen shirts.

The publication of *The Poor and the Poorest*, by highlighting the importance of the concept of relative poverty in Britain at large, led to further research into the living conditions of the poor and their health status when compared with those who were better off. In Scotland, in 1975, the Chief Medical of Health for Scotland Sir John Brotherston, in his Galton Lecture, expressed the concern of many working in the NHS who had called attention to the social gulf which existed in health. He did so by giving statistics from the Scottish Registrar General's data and from the English Central Statistical Office.

He commenced his Galton Lecture thus:

> There is so much evidence demonstrating differences in mortality and morbidity between the social classes as defined by our Registrars General that it is difficult to select from the evidence. I demonstrate them here in terms of total mortality experience for adults. I demostrate also differences in experience in maternity and infancy.

These social class differences are not limited to mortality and morbidity. They run through the whole gamut of physical attributes upon which estimates are made of normal health development – for example, there are differences in birth weights and persisting differences in height and weight of school children in different social classes.

Table 11.1 Male standardised mortality ratios: by social class (England and Wales)

Social Class	1921–3 (age 20–64)	1930–2 (age 20–64)	1949–53 (age 20–64)	1959–63 (age 15–64)	1970–2 (age 15–64)
I	82	90	86	76	77
II	94	94	92	81	81
III	95	97	101	100	104
IV	101	102	104	103	113
V	125	111	118	143	137

Source: Central Statistical Office (1975) The table sources are marked as 1921–63 RGs Decennial Supplements: Occupational Mortality 1951 and 1961, 1970–72, Office of Population Census and Surveys.* i.e. the 1970–72 figures are marked 'Provisional data'.

In England, the Department of Health and Social Security had been expressing concern with Britain's failure to match the improvements in health in some other advanced countries, and had acknowledged some relationship between this and persistent inequalities of health (DHSS 1976). But it was not until 1977, in a speech on 27 March, that David Ennals, then the Labour Secretary of State for Social Services, said:

> the crude differences in mortality rates between the various social classes are worrying. To take the extreme example, in 1971 the death rate for adult men in social class V (unskilled workers) was nearly twice that of adult men in social class I (professional workers). ... when you look at death rates for specific diseases the gap is even wider .... The first step towards remedial action is to put together what is already known about the problem ... it is a major challenge for the next ten or more years to try to narrow the gap in health standards between different social classes.
>
> (Whitehead 1992)

Table 11.2 Infant mortality rates per 1,000 live births by social class for Scotland (1961 and 1970)

Social class	1961	1970	Per cent decrease 1961–70
I and II	17.4	12.0	31
III	25.1	18.6	26
IV and V	30.0	25.4	15
IV and V as a percentage of I and II	172.0	212.0	

Source: Scottish Registrar General's Data (1961 and 1970).

Table 11.3   Health defects in school children, 1973

Social class of parent	Scotland					
	Percentages of school children at the age of 5 suffering from				Height of school children at the age of 14 (cm)	
	Uncorrected refractive error in eyesight		Dental caries			
	Boys	Girls	Boys	Girls	Boys	Girls
I	3.7	2.9	6.7	8.2	158	156
II	3.6	5.4	8.3	9.4	156	156
III	4.6	4.6	14.5	15.7	155	155
IV	5.1	6.2	16.7	19.7	154	154
V	8.6	7.8	21.2	20.6	152	153
All classes	5.0	5.3	20.6	16.6	154	154

Source: Scottish Information Services Division (Brotherston 1975)

Accordingly in April 1977 a Working Group was set up by David Ennals with the following terms of reference:

(1) To assemble available information about the differences in health status among the social classes and about factors which might contribute to these, including relevant data from other industrial countries; (2) To analyse this material in order to identify possible causal relationships, to examine the hypotheses that have been formulated and the testing of them, to assess the implications for policy; and (3) To suggest what further research should be initiated.

(*ibid.*: xi)

The members of the Working Group included Sir Douglas Black (Chairman), Chief Scientist at the Department of Health and Social Security and President of the Royal College of Physicians, and Professor Peter Townsend, Professor of Social Policy, University of Bristol. The report was known as the 'Black Report' after its Chairman (a Scot). It was submitted to the Secretary of State of the new Conservative administration in April 1980 and received a 'frosty' reception. Its main findings were that the poorer health of the lower occupational groups applied at all stages of life. Further:

The class gradient seemed to be greater than in some comparable countries ... and was becoming more marked. During the twenty years up to the early 1970s covered by the Black Report, the mortality rates for both men and women aged 35 and over in occupational classes I and II had steadily diminished while those in IV and V changed very little *or had deteriorated.*

(*ibid.*: 2)

The Working Group argued that the main problem lay outside the NHS and that socio-economic factors, such as income, employment (or unemployment), education, housing, transport and 'lifestyles' all affected health in favour of those who were better off. There were two main policy thrusts: 'one calling for a total and not merely a service-oriented approach to the problems of health; and two, calling for a radical overhaul of the balance of activity and proportionate distribution of resources within the health and associated services' (Whitehead 1992: 3).

The 'frosty' response from the government was encapsulated in the Foreword to the Report by Patrick Jenkin, the new Conservative Secretary of State for Social Services, when he wrote:

It will come as a disappointment to many that over long periods since the inception of the National Health Service there is generally little sign of health inequalities in Britain actually diminishing and, in some cases, they may be increasing .... I must make it clear that additional expenditure on the scale which could result from the report's recommendations – the amount involved could be upwards of £2 billion a year – is quite unrealistic in present or any foreseeable economic circumstances.

(*ibid.*: 33 Foreword)

Thus, although there was overwhelming evidence that there is a health divide between the rich and the poor in the United Kingdom, nothing was done at a national level, although there were examples of action at local level in Birmingham City and Strathclyde Region (see later).

The next significant move at national level was in 1986 when the Health Education Council commissioned Margaret Whitehead to update the evidence on inequalities and health that had accumulated since 1980, and to assess the progress made on the thirty-seven recommendations of the Black Report. The publication and launch of this new report, *The Health Divide*, on 24 March 1987, received a mixed reception, partly because it was seen by the Chairman of the Health Education Council, Sir Brian Bailey, as 'political dynamite in an election year' (*The Independent* 25 March 1987).

This report essentially repeated the main findings of the Black Report, but showed that inequalities in health were widening and that the poor were getting sicker in relative terms. Because of the uproar created upon its publication *The Health Divide* was read by a much wider audience than expected and, in the House of Commons, a debate on social and economic inequalities (6 April 1987) gave a great deal of prominence to the findings of the book on health inequalities. Twenty-six MPs put down a Commons motion calling for a programme which recognised the relationship between poverty and poor health. *The Health Divide* also provoked a series of partisan responses by politicians designed to discredit the book's findings and that of the Black Report, by suggesting they were politically biased and did not reflect mainstream scientific opinion. Thus, during the Commons debate, Mr Ray Whitney, Conservative MP and former Under-Secretary of State for Health stated:

> These issues can be approached from a class bias, a fascination with a class division of society which is basically a Marxist approach .... Marxism is entirely based on this class approach and is carefully reflected in the 'Black Report' and *The Health Divide*.
>
> (House of Commons 1987)

Some of the MPs on the opposition benches reminded the former minister that the Archbishop of Canterbury's commission on *Faith in the City* had likewise been labelled Marxist when it raised the issues of poverty and deprivation in the cities. Among the press, which reported *The Health Divide* very widely (it was front-page news in all the national press, tabloid and broadsheet), the *News of the World* saw more sinister undertones and went so far as to suggest that the whole affair was part of a plot by an anti-government group ('reds') to 'hijack' the Health Education Council. The original Preface to *The Health Divide* stirred strong reaction – favourable and otherwise:

> This final report from the Health Education Council before its demise on 31 March 1987 is, in my opinion, an essential element in the public debate which must occur on health inequalities in the United Kingdom. Such inequality is inexcusable in a democratic society which prides itself on being humane. To eliminate or even reduce it substantially would be a major contribution to the health of the people of this country.
>
> (*ibid.*: 290–1)

The Black Report and *The Health Divide* also showed a divide in rates of illness and death between nations and regions in the United Kingdom. Thus the healthiest part of the United Kingdom appears to have been the southern belt below a line drawn from the Wash to the Bristol Channel, while the highest morbidity and mortality rates were in the poorest parts of the United Kingdom, that is, Scotland and the northern region of England. Scotland had the second-highest death rates in the world in men, from coronary heart disease and lung cancer; in women it had the highest death rates in the world from lung cancer. A conflating factor in coronary heart disease and lung cancer is the smoking of cigarettes; smoking is directly related to social class with social class V males and females smoking almost twice as much as social class I.

It had been known for some time that mortality within the United Kingdom differed, with England having the lowest and Scotland and Northern Ireland the highest mortality rates. In 1989 Carstairs and Morris published a paper in the *British Medical Journal* entitled: 'Deprivation: Explaining Differences in Mortality between Scotland and England and Wales'. They demonstrated that deprivation was much more severe in Scotland, and was related to mortality, with gradients being particularly strong in young adults. The following tables taken from this paper clearly illustrate the facts.

The findings of *The Health Divide* deserve more detailed scrutiny. The pattern showed that serious and persisting social inequalities in health were found on many fronts.

The picture emerges of those at the bottom of the social scale, however measured, having much poorer health and survival chances. Using *occupational class* as an indicator of social position, then the poorer health of the socially disadvantaged shows up not only in mortality statistics but also in morbidity figures and, most recently, in new indicators of positive health and well-being. It is apparent for most causes of death and also for the major diseases which are chronic and painful, but not life threatening, such as arthritis. Such inequalities in health are not limited to one period in life but are evident from infancy to old age.

There are some problems with using occupational class, but if the results are checked against other measures like *housing tenure* or *car ownership*, a consistent pattern of inequality is still seen. The Black Report documented a clear

Table 11.4 Proportion (%) of population * living at differing categories of deprivation (Scotland and England and Wales)

Deprivation score	Deprivation category †	Scotland	England and Wales
<−1.4−	1	6.1	23.8
−1.4−	2	13.7	30.4
−0.8−	3	21.8	21.5
−0.3−	4	25.5	14.1
0.3−	5	14.8	6.7
0.8−	6	11.4	2.9
>1.7	7	6.8	0.5

* Population of Scotland 5,035,000; England and Wales 48,552,000.
† 1 = affluent, 7 = deprived.

Table 11.5   Social class distributions (%), Scotland and England and Wales *Population* *

Social class	Men aged 20–64		Women aged 20–64	
	Scotland	England and Wales	Scotland	England and Wales
I	5.4	5.6	4.5	4.5
II	19.1	21.9	14.9	19.1
III (Non-manual)	9.9	10.8	8.8	9.2
III (Manual)	36.3	33.4	28.1	26.1
IV	17.1	15.3	12.8	12.1
V	7.3	5.5	5.2	4.0
In forces or inadequately described	4.9	3.0	2.4	2.4
Not economically active	3.6	4.4	22.7	23.5

*Population in households with head in social class stated and economically active. Population figures: men in Scotland 1,382,000; England and Wales 13,634,000. Population in Scotland 5,035,000. England and Wales 48,552,000.

Table 11.6   Mortality (per 1,000 population) for Scotland and England and Wales, 1980–2

I Age (years)	Scotland		England and Wales	
	M	F	M	F
0-	3.3	2.5	3.1	2.4
5-	0.3	0.2	0.3	0.2
15-	1.0	0.3	0.8	0.3
25-	1.1	0.6	0.9	0.5
35-	2.6	1.6	1.8	1.3
45-	8.0	4.9	6.1	3.7
55-	21.9	12.3	17.7	9.6
65-	53.2	30.2	48.1	25.2
>_75	134.9	99.1	122.5	90.3

pattern of higher mortality in the North and West of the Country and lower mortality in the South and East in the 1970s. This North/South divide was still just as evident in the 1980s. For example, death rates among both men and women of working age are close to twice as high on Clydeside as in East Anglia. So it appears that there is a clear North/South divide in health. But what is its significance? In the past ten years or so many studies have been carried out to look at the health profiles of much smaller areas than those of Regions or Health Authorities. These *small area studies* reveal a much more complex picture. They find that communities living side by side in the same region can have widely different health profiles, with pockets of very poor health alongside pockets of much better health. This led Greater Glasgow Health Board to report: 'In several communities (in Glasgow) death rates were as low (or lower) than in the healthiest countries in the world whereas in many others death rates are among the highest anywhere'

A very detailed study in Sheffield (Thunhurst 1985) reached similar conclusions: a difference of over eight years in life expectancy for men between the best and worst wards.

These pockets of poor health corresponded to areas of poverty and material deprivation, while the pockets of better health correspond to more affluent areas. In the Northern Regional Health Authority, 65 per cent of the difference in health between wards could be 'explained' statistically by deprivation indicators (Thunhurst 1985: 248).

Another important finding is that there are healthy wards in the Northern Region (North East of England around Newcastle), which compare favourably with the healthier wards in the South (around Bristol) and vice versa. Thus, on closer inspection, the North/South health divide appears to be more a deprived/affluent health divide, with the poorer health profile of the North overall reflecting the greater concentration of deprivation in that area.

The health of the population as a whole has continued to improve over the past decade – if measured by death rates, life expectancy, height, dental health, etc. In fact mortality has been declining all this century. But have these improvements been experienced equally across all sections of the community or have some benefited more than others? Are some lagging behind? Is the health gap getting wider, narrower, or is it about the same? The Black Report reviewed evidence from 1931 to 1971 and concluded that the gap in health between the advantaged and disadvantaged had in some cases stayed the same, while in others it had become *wider*. What has happened in the decades from 1971? Certainly, in adults of working age, non-manual groups experienced a faster decline in death rates than manual groups, so the health gap widened. In some of the major killers, death rates *increased* for the manual classes while showing a *decline* in non-manual classes: for example, a 1 per cent increase in mortality in male manual workers and a 15 per cent decrease for male non-manual workers. In women, lung cancer and CHD mortality increased in manual classes, while decreasing in non-manual classes. In babies at birth and in the first month of life, the health gap stayed the same, but for post-neonatal mortality the health gap decreased – a very welcome trend

For older people after the age of 65 (when most deaths now occur), we do not have information on mortality trends *yet*, but the Office of Population Censuses and Surveys Longitudinal Study has shown that previous occupation is still a powerful indicator of the risk of death after 65, and after 75 for that matter (*ibid.*: 233).

Trends in *morbidity* from 1974 show an *increase* in rates of reported illness (unlike death rates, which are declining). Illness rates in manual groups have consistently been higher than in non-manual groups over the period 1974–84, and the gap between the two has increased over that time, particularly in the over-65 age group.

Similar trends are found using other indicators: from 1971 to 1981 there was a decline in mortality for degree-holders, while there was no decline for those with no educational qualifications.

There are many problems with tracing longer-term health trends, but there have been three re-analyses of the data from 1921 to 1971, which basically concluded that all classes have profited from the decline in mortality but higher-status groups have profited more than most. The conclusion from the most recent evidence is still in line with that of the Black Report in 1980: socio-economic factors (including lifestyles) play the major part in maintaining inequalities in health.

The way ahead

Since the publication of the Black Report and *The Health Divide*, research has continued. Pressure groups such as the Child Poverty Action Group, the Low-Pay Unit and the Public Health Alliance have been set up, and local and national initiatives have spread. With regard to research, two most relevant and important works have been *Unfair Shares: The Effects of Widening Income Differences on the Welfare of the Young* by Richard Wilkinson, published by Barnardo's in 1994, and the *Inquiry into Income and Wealth* published by the Joseph Rowntree Foundation in February 1995. The first, *Unfair Shares* has made a powerful impact on the media, and it is worth quoting here as an example *The Guardian* editorial of 28 July 1994:

> Every prophet needs a bible: and Barnardo's has thoughtfully provided Labour's latest prophet with a new testament. Its message … could not be more challenging: relative poverty is even more corrosive of health, emotional welfare and social behaviour than absolute poverty …
>
> The basic facts are familiar: inequality in the UK has grown faster and wider in the last decade than in any previous period since records began over 100 years ago …

What is new is just how devastating relative poverty has become ... the pamphlet is filled with correlation charts showing the slowing down of declining death (and sickness) rates for infants, children and young adults, with a corresponding increase in inequality ...

The second report, the *Inquiry into Income and Wealth* was equally powerful and its findings were similar to those of *Unfair Shares*.

As far as the pressure groups are concerned, as well as intensive parliamentary lobbying they organise conferences and produce a variety of publications. Two worth mentioning are *Poverty: The Facts* (Oppenheim 1990), published by the Child Poverty Action Group and The Low-Pay Unit's *The Virus that Affects Us All* (Player 1993) published in *The New Review*.

In respect of local and national initiatives, an example of a local initiative in Birmingham, which has now been taken up in Edinburgh and Fife, is described in 'Citizens' Advice in General Practice' (Paris and Player 1993). An example of a national initiative is the production of a Poverty and Health Resource pack entitled *Poverty and Health: Tools for Change* by the Public Health Alliance (1995). This resource was launched in London on 24 April 1995 at the offices of the Association of Metropolitan Authorities and further launches and workshops were held throughout May 1995 in Belfast, Glasgow, Birmingham and Liverpool, supported by the Northern Ireland Health Promotion Agency, Glasgow Healthy Cities Project, Greater Glasgow Health Board, Healthy Birmingham 2000, Health Promotion Wales, Liverpool City Council and Barnsley Community Health Council.

Throughout the 1980s and 1990s, Scotland offered many examples of resistance to policies which might degrade public health. The referendum on water privatisation organised by Strathclyde Region produced a huge affirmation of support for publicly owned water services. The late 1990s also saw the resurgence of a number of anti-poverty campaigns. One such campaign centred on the abolition of Scotland's system of poindings and warrant sales.

Poindings and warrant sales are a pernicious and degrading form of debt recovery, established under Scots law several centuries ago and used extensively in the highland clearances. They involve sheriff's officers poinding, that is laying legal claim, to a debtor's household goods, for a subsequent public auction known as a warrant sale. The process, done in full public view, is humiliating and has resonances of the Poor Law mentality that many Scots had been fighting throughout the century.

Another campaign sought to combat food poverty, especially among children, through pressure to introduce free fruit, free breakfasts and free school meals for all school children.

By 1999 Scotland had a very specific institution to which these issues could be addressed and from whom solutions and action could be sought, the Scottish Parliament. The constitutional constraints referred to by Brotherston at the beginning of this chapter could now (at least in part) be removed by a Parliament with authority over health, housing and education.

The breach created in 1707 which Brotherston claims had served Scotland so ill, was closed when presiding officer Winnie Ewing uttered the momentous words:

> This Parliament is reconvened.

Many in Scotland felt that this would portend new strides in combating poverty and inequalities in health. It was after all a famous German physician of social medicine, Rudolf Virchow, who said in the early part of the twentieth century that:

> Medicine is a social science and politics nothing but medicine on a grand scale.

> (Rosen 1974)

Conclusions

Several conclusions can be drawn from an historical overview of poverty in Scotland and the effects of poverty on the health of the poor and, indeed, the health of the nation as a whole. Scotland entered the century benefiting from the advances in public health practice, water systems, sewerage, etc. of the previous century, but with little concern to improve the lot of the poor.

It took the impact of the Boer War and then the First World War, the exposure of the housing and general living conditions of the poor, who were dying in their tens of thousands in Flanders and France, to impel the government of Lloyd George to speak of 'homes fit for heroes'. Although the inter-war period did not see decisively effective action, the issue was firmly on the agenda.

But it was the Second World War and the politicisation of the British people for democracy and against fascism which brought the concept of a welfare state nearer to implementation. The impact of the Beveridge Report in 1942, aimed against the five giants of Want, Ignorance, Sickness, Squalor and Idleness, had an impact which has not disappeared. The general election of 1945 and a Labour government with a sizeable working majority made the implementation of the welfare state a reality, despite the dire economic position. The crucial factor was that the 'will' was there.

The NHS, introduced in Scotland and England on 5 July 1948, was seen by most people as the epitome of the welfare state, and has remained so until the present day. The condition of the poor, however, was not changed overnight and the optimism in this area was dashed by the publication on Christmas Eve 1965 of *The Poor and the Poorest* by Townsend and Abel-Smith. This was a watershed in the approach to poverty in Britain, for it re-introduced the concepts of absolute and relative poverty and described how the numbers living in relative poverty were in fact increasing. Subsequent reports such as the Black Report and *The Health Divide* in 1980 and 1987 respectively, showed that the gap between the rich and the poor was increasing in financial and in health terms. This became increasingly unacceptable in countries such as Scotland and England, which liked to consider themselves civilised. The more recent work on this subject by Wilkinson, *Unfair Shares: The Effects of Widening Income Differences on the Welfare of the Young* published by Barnardo's in 1994, showed that Scotland, England and the United States of America are lagging behind other advanced industrial countries in terms of income distribution and the overall health of their peoples. The message is clear. Over 400 years ago the Elizabethan philosopher and poet Sir Francis Bacon (1561–1626) said in his *Essays, Civil and Moral*: 'Of great riches there is no real use, except it be in the distribution.'

Scotland's own poet had perhaps the last word on the subject and it was appropriate that these words were sung at the official opening of the Scottish Parliament in 1999:

> Then let us pray that come it may
> (As come it will for a' that)
> That Sense and Worth o'er a' the earth
> Shall bear the gree an' a' that!
> For a' that, an' a' that,
> It's comin yet for a' that,
> That man to man the world o'er
> Shall brithers be for a' that.

References

Bevan, A. (1952) 'In Place of Fear', London: Heinemann, pp. 81, 85.

Brotherston, J. (1975) 'Inequality: Is it Inevitable?', the Galton Lecture, in C.O. Carter and J. Peel (eds) *Equalities and Inequalities in Health*. London: Academic Press, pp. 73–6.

Brotherston, J. (1987) 'Introduction', in G. McLachlan, *Improving the Common Weal: Aspects of Scottish Health Services 1900–1984*. Edinburgh: Edinburgh University Press.

Brown, G. and Cook, R. (eds) (1983) 'The Historical Background', in *Scotland: The Real Divide*. Edinburgh: Mainstream, pp. 66–9.

Carstairs, V. and Morris, R. (1989) 'Deprivation: Explaining Differences in Mortality between Scotland and England and Wales', *British Medical Journal* 299: 886–9.

Department of Health and Social Security (DHSS) (1976)*Prevention and Health: Everybody's Business*. London: HMSO.

Department of Health for Scotland (1936) *Report of the Committee on Scottish Health Services* (Cathcart Report), Cmnd 5402. Edinburgh.

Department of Health for Scotland (1944) *Report for the Year Ended 30.6.1945*, Cmnd 6502. London.

Greater Glasgow Health Board (1984) *Ten Year Report, 1974–1983*. Glasgow: .

Harvie, C. (1981) *No Gods and Precious Few Heroes: Scotland 1914–1980*. London: Edward Arnold.

HMSO (1942) *Social Insurance and Allied Services* (Beveridge Report), Cmnd 6404. London: HMSO.

House of Commons Debates – 6 April 1987.

Joseph Rowntree Foundation (1995) *Inquiry into Income and Wealth*, 2 vols. York: Joseph Rowntree Foundation.

Lowe, R. (1993) *The Welfare State in Britain Since 1945*. London: Macmillan.

Mackintosh, J.M. (1953) *Trends of Opinion about the Public Health 1901–1951*. Oxford.

McLachlan, G. (ed.) (1987) *Improving the Common Weal: Aspects of Scottish Health Services 1900–1984*. Edinburgh: Edinburgh University Press.

MacNalty, A.S. (ed.) (1955) *History of the Second World War*, UK Medical Series, Civilian Health and Medical Services, vol. 2. London.

Oppenheim, C. (1990) *Poverty: The Facts*. London: Child Poverty Action Group.

Paris, J.A. and Player, D.A. (1993) 'Citizens' Advice in General Practice', *British Medical Journal* 306: 1518–20.

'Parliamentary Debates: Official Report' – Fifth Series 14 July 1936, vol. 314, col. 1905.

Player, D.A. (1993) 'The Virus that Affects Us All', *The New Review* (Low-Pay Unit) October/November.

Public Health Alliance (PHA) (1995) *Poverty and Health: Tools for Change*. Birmingham: PHA.

Rosen, G. (1974) 'What is Social Medicine?' in G. Rosen (ed.) *From Medical Police to Social Medicine: Essays on the History of Health Care*. New York: Science History Publications.

Smith, A. (1812) *An Enquiry into the Natural Causes of the Wealth of Nations*. London:

Thunhurst, C. (1985) *Poverty and Health in the City of Sheffield*. Sheffield: City Council Environmental Health Department.

Whitehead, M. (1992)'The Health Divide', in P. Townsend, M. Whitehead and N. Davidson *Inequalities in Health*, new edn. Harmondsworth: Penguin.

Wilkinson, R. (1994) *Unfair Shares: The Effects of Widening Income Differences on the Welfare of the Young. Environmental Health Department*. Ilford: Barnardo's.

Chapter 12

Valuing 'lay' and practitioner knowledge in evaluation

The role of participatory evaluation in health promotion

Jane Springett

Introduction

The future of health promotion and our greater understanding of its social significance depends on the development of its knowledge base. How that knowledge base is developed is dependent on adopting approaches to evaluation that are consistent with the values and principles underpinning health promotion and which acknowledge as well as capture its social implications. The recent nature of the health promotion field, the relative underfunding of health promotion research compared with biomedicine and disease prevention, and the reluctance, in the past, of practitioners to evaluate what they are trying to achieve in a systematic way means that our knowledge base is relatively limited (South and Tilford 2000). It is limited too, by an over-concern with 'objective evidence' which ignores the unique knowledge and experience of ordinary people and those working in the field (Everitt 1996). Evaluation is more than collecting evidence, it is about knowledge development and critical praxis.

Health promotion involves changing the power relations so excluded groups can have a say and 'take control' of the factors that create health (Labonte 1994, 1999). The most appropriate type of evaluation, therefore, is one that involves enhancing this control. Making explicit who the evaluation is for is the first stage in addressing issues of oppression. However, there is a need to go beyond that. Being true to the central tenets of health promotion means an appropriate approach to evaluation is one that does not, at the very minimum, contribute to disempowerment but at best empowers.

This chapter will focus on participatory evaluation which aims to do that. Participatory evaluation is an approach to evaluation, not a method. It will be argued that participatory evaluation is most in keeping in its approach with the values of health promotion. Moreover it is the approach to evaluation that is most likely to contribute to learning and knowledge development within the practice of health promotion.

The influence of disease prevention traditions on health promotion evaluation

Essentially, evaluation is a process by which you judge whether something is worth doing and whereby an assessment is made as to the value of certain actions. Evaluation is something we do naturally all the time. It is a process of reflection. It is also a process of learning from experience and a potential vehicle for informal and life-long learning (Brown *et al.* 1995; Watkins and Marsik 1992). Some distinguish one type of evaluation from another in terms of method or technique, but method should not drive an evaluation (Pawson and Tilley 1998). Much more important is the evaluation question, which flows from the purpose of the evaluation. For example, is the purpose to find out if community needs are met, to improve the intervention or programme, to assess its outcomes, to find out how it is operating, to assess the efficiency, or to understand why a programme of innovation works or does not work? Each of these questions may differ depending on the nature of the health promotion initiative and on the context. It is questions like these that are crucial for the development of the field of health promotion, so more is known about what works and, more importantly, why and in what context.

Evaluation is different from formal research. While it often uses the techniques and tools of research, it differs in a number of important ways. A key difference lies within the word itself, the notion of value and its assessment. While it is widely recognised, in social science at least, that research is not value free, the conventions of science attempt to limit, through a variety of checks and balances, the degree of deviation from so-called 'objectivity'. By contrast, value lies at the centre of evaluation. It always has a political dimension and is intimately tied up with societal priorities, resource allocation and power (Greene 1994). At the heart of evaluation, the question has to be asked whose values are driving the evaluation, and by whose standards are the activities being undertaken and assessed, or being measured against? For health promotion interventions this raises important issues, as quite often the values against which they are being assessed are not those of the field or the people with whom health promoters are working but those of a dominant ideology (Springett 2001).

Historically this has certainly been the case. The dominance and power of medicine in health and the consequential sanctity of the Randomised Controlled Trial, traditional epidemiology and the conventional scientific method, based as it is in a positivist epistemology, has had a great influence on what research and evaluation has been funded and what is published in scientific journals. Disease prevention continues to dominate the agenda. In disease prevention, underpinned as it is by the medical model, the primary focus is not on the person but on a single disease as a problem, with a specific aetiology and pathology. Population health is seen as the aggregate of the risk behaviour of individuals. The intention behind any action or intervention is on the negative – stopping something happening – rather than encouraging something to develop or change. The focus of interest, for example diabetes or heart disease, as well as the nature of any intervention, is determined primarily by the expert opinion that defined the 'health state' in the first place. On the whole the 'lay' perspective is not valued or at best lip-service is paid to it (Williams and Popay 1994). Moreover, a linear causal mechanism is understood to underpin the intervention, with a clear relationship between intervention input and outcome. 'Success' is defined as not dying (mortality) or not experiencing the disease (morbidity) or, more often, a reduction in the demand for specific medical interventions or in the demand for hospital beds. The concern is with the individual rather than the individual in his or her social context and each individual is expected to be treated largely as the same. Also the source of the problem and the solution is considered to be primarily physical even if it is located externally, such as in the environment (pollution) and/or behavioural (poor diet) or, as often in practice, to a chemical imbalance and the need for a drug.

This perspective is reflected in the language of evaluation as applied to disease prevention interventions. The intervention is characterised as treatment and the nature of that treatment as a dose (Chen 1990). The outcome is a single state too; the only change is that which takes place between the start of the intervention and the end. Thus evaluation frameworks call for pre-test and post-test data-collection points (Shephard 1996). Context is deemed as given and unchanging during the operation of the 'experiment'. Thus the focus is on objective measurement, the primacy of control and compliance, on hierarchy, separation of mind and emotion from body, and spirit from either. Such types of evaluation are clearly located in a Cartesian paradigm of science. Descartes emphasised dualism, reductionism, separateness – the primacy of the rational and logical over feeling, and objective measurement over subjective experience. For the Cartesian, only that which is measurable exists and counts as evidence. As a result what is measurable is made important, since method drives the way the intervention is evaluated. However, the measurements that result are often meaningless in relation to the social reality of people's lives, where social relationships, feelings and intuition are important. The reverence given to the primacy of a particular form of science that is the historical baggage of disease prevention limits what is looked at to only a small segment of reality. Not only is the glass half empty, but also only one segment of the glass is seen and deemed to exist.

Health, according to the *Ottawa Charter*, is created in everyday life through the way people work; play and love (WHO 1986). In other words, it is socially constructed. Health promotion also usually involves some form of social interaction and the development of human relationships. Increasingly, there is a consensus that 'good' health promotion necessarily involves engaging people in the process (Labonte 1999; Wallerstein and Freudenberg 1998). This applies to most health promotion as praxis, whether it still is aimed at individual behavioural change or, as is increasingly the case, on action focused on the broader social determinants of health (Frankish *et al.* 1998). Underpinning the ideology of health promotion there is also a basic concern for social justice. This focus on people rather than on risk factors is encapsulated in Raeburn and Rootman's notion of people-centred health promotion (1998). They argue that such an approach must start from people's own experience and be grounded in everyday reality rather than an artificial 'setting'. The professional involved should see themselves as a facil-itator of change with a focus on strength building while respecting and honouring the individual and the developmental process. The focus is on positive change.

Since health promotion is fundamentally a social process (Nutbeam 1998) it does not involve a single act followed by a clear outcome that is fixed in space and time. The boundary between the 'intervention' and the social process or context into which it is intervening is often blurred. Everything is constantly in a state of flux. In good community-based health promotion the nature of the action taken will evolve as understanding among all partic-ipants changes, particularly where the initial concerns are defined by the community and not the health sector agency. Indeed, one could characterise health promotion as a decision making process involving a number of key agents whose actions contribute in varying degrees to the final outcome. The individual decision makers can be organisations or individuals, none of whom operate in a vacuum but in an environment created by other members in the process, so the process is a complex circular one of constant inter-action. Each participant can initiate or veto the change favoured by others, but any innovation is taking place in the broader context established by others. This is in essence a whole-systems or ecological approach to popula-tion health, where the emphasis is on the relationship between the individual and the environment (Glouberman 2000).

By implication, too, health promotion also requires a consistency in the application of change processes over a period of time and at a number of levels. In the promotion of health, we are looking at complex social phenomena requiring complex interventions. Those interventions may take the form of a project or programme but equally could take the form of a policy or an innovative social change. There is no magic bullet with health promotion. There are in fact multiple strategies and multiple outcomes, some intended and some not. There is also no clear linear relationship between input and outcome. Outcome is usually the product of a complex interaction between factors including context. Everything changes, including the perceptions of those involved as to what is important and the meanings given to actions and events (Van Eyk *et al.* 2001). In this interactive flux new knowledge is created. That new knowledge cannot be captured and devel-oped through old experimental and positivist approaches to evaluation. What is required is the development and use of evaluation approaches that acknowledge the complexity and give voice to many different forms of knowledge and, most importantly, through their practice empower people to act on the knowledge they have played a part in developing.

Knowledge development for health promotion

Traditional methods driven evaluation embedded in positivist science creates an exclusive form of knowledge and knowledge development. Essentially elitist, only certain forms of knowledge are valued. Quantitative information is consistently given primacy over qualitative and 'expert' over 'lay' and popular knowledge (Garanta 1993). The day-to-day experience of practitioners too is considered inferior and largely irrelevant. In many of the published evaluations that appear in academic journals, the focus of the evaluation question and the intervention that is being evaluated is largely derived from the narrow research interests of a group of researchers and their peer groups. Moreover, there is little emphasis on making a contribution to the intervention or project while it is under way. Dissemination is seen as a key to future change, most commonly through a research paper or perhaps through a research seminar. On the whole research and development are kept separate (Peile 1994). Changes to practice are expected to take place automatically after the dissemination process, because it is expected that the practitioner, now equipped with the new research knowledge, will incorporate it into their work in the form of evidence-based practice. In reality this rarely happens. The findings of research may not resonate with the practitioner's experience because the context is so different. Or, as is more often the case, the focus on outcomes means very little is reported on the actual process (of implementation). Sometimes practitioners will implement an approach which is reported as being, for example, 80 per cent effective in a controlled study, and find it ineffective. For, as Kushner (2000) has argued, evidence-based practice is often the fossilisation of practical ideas into context-less formulae which do not work.

Nowhere is this more apparent than in the area of smoking cessation interventions in the UK. The initial intervention that received government funding was a free one-week supply of Nicotell(tm) patches. The intervention was based on a meta-analysis of the published literature against the gold standard criteria of the RCT, which established that was the most effective and, particularly, cost effective intervention. Underpinning the rationale was the view that poor people would choose to take the free Nicotell patches and from the money saved through not buying cigarettes in the first week, would fund their subsequent supply of patches (Lake and Wood 2000). However, research has demonstrated that such an approach depends on context, both the economic context and the socio-cultural context, particularly the role cigarettes play in people's everyday lives, suggesting that effective intervention will be more variable in space and time (Graham 1998; Wood *et al.* in press).

Even in the field of evaluation, as opposed to research, the new knowledge created through traditional evaluation is rarely utilised (Weiss 1988). Here the focus historically has been on producing a report for funders and managers at the conclusion of an evaluation. The executive summary is read and then the report placed on a shelf to collect dust, the knowledge created confined to a select and powerful few, rarely shared with the community as a whole and equally rarely acted upon. These conventional approaches also reinforce the marginalisation of the least powerful. Problems are often seen to be located in a particular community or a particular ethnic group, and both the evaluation and the intervention often focus exclusively on that community, rather than on the context in which those groups operate (Goodman *et al.* 1995). Little is done in the evaluation process to probe the experience and assumptions of the organisations that are the source of disempowerment, or to bring the two groups together in a dialogue concerning the problem, the programme, and how its success/failure will be evaluated and against whose criteria. As a result, little is learnt about the power structures and conflicts that people experience, or how the barriers to structural change might be overcome.

Furthermore, knowledge creation is more than knowing the facts, it is about integrating that knowledge and being aware of how it can be used in different circumstances. It is about learning and learning for change. It is both a social and an individual process (Cranton 1996). Learning can be understood as 'a self-regulated process of resolving inner cognitive conflicts that often become apparent through concrete experience, collaborative discourse and reflection' (Brooks and Brooks 1993: viii). Kolb (1984) in his model of the adult experiential learning cycle argues that, for learning to take place, all elements of the cycle of thinking, deciding, doing and reflecting must be accomplished. There is an intrinsic connection, therefore, between knowledge and action. What people do is absolutely bound up with what they know and think, and what they know and think is bound up with what they do. Most people adopt new information only when it conforms to their pre-existing view of the world. Transformation comes through critical engagement with, and reflection on, the issues, and through what Freire (1976) called the process of *conscientisation*. Participation at all stages of an evaluation by all those who are involved in the outcomes of an intervention or programme or policy would therefore appear to be funda-mental to this learning process. Nor should this participation be confined to those with power such as funding bodies and managers. If health promo-tion is about social relations and, more particularly, about helping the more marginalised in society, and if it is about encouraging the development of social structures that create health, then community and practitioner involvement should underpin the evaluation of health promotion and its knowledge construction. The evaluation then becomes health promoting in itself.

The nature of participatory approaches to evaluation

Participatory approaches to evaluation are those which attempt to involve in an evaluation all who have a stake in its outcomes, with a view to taking action and effecting change (Springett 2001). As has been argued above, if evaluation is going to change anything it has to be useful and perceived as useful by those involved in a project or programme, whether as a funder, a participant or project worker. All are experts in terms of different forms of knowledge about the programme project or policy concerned. External evaluators also add their expertise. Each participant has something to teach the others and something to learn from the others, creating a series of teacher–learner cycles (Pawson and Tilley 1998). In answering different sets of questions at different stages of the evaluation process different teacher–learner cycles are set up. The aim should be to maximise the knowledge and learning generated through such cycles.

The aim with participatory evaluation is an approach that encourages every voice to be heard and, at the very least, taken into consideration when deciding on the focus and design of the evaluation (Fawcett *et al* 2001). Participatory evaluation, however, goes beyond just being aware of stakeholder interests, in that there is a joint responsibility for the evaluation by the participants who also play an active role in the nuts and bolts of evaluation (Cousins and Earl 1995; Robson 2000). In participatory evaluation the focus is on knowledge creation in the context of practice to encourage the development of local theory and capacity to build, and to encourage local learning and development (Garanta 1993). Such a perspective is based on a completely different conception of the relationship between science, knowledge, learning and action than is found in positivist methods in social science. It assumes that people can generate knowledge as partners in a systematic inquiry process based on their own categories and frameworks. It creates active support for the results of the process of inquiry, and therefore greater commitment to change as well as greater likelihood that ideas will be diffused and more people will learn from them (Gustavsen 1992). The aim of participatory evaluation is to make change, and teach a self-generating and self-maintaining process which continues after the evaluator/researcher has left. The essence of this type of evaluation is that it is an emergent process controlled by local conditions (Wallerstein 1999). Participatory evaluation is potentially empowering. It encourages innovation and change. This is in contrast to traditional approaches to evaluation, which can easily undermine innovation. As people become aware of being judged, they perform to satisfy the measurement chosen instead of improving capability. The intrinsic motivation that drives learning and creates change is replaced by a desire to provide numbers for bureaucrats (Henkel 1991; Seddon 2000).

The strength of participatory evaluation is that it integrates evaluation into project work allowing a more naturally emerging and evolving approach to the development of aims and objectives (Springett and Leavey 1995). It is not outcomes driven. Rather it is plays a key role in consciousness raising. In particular, it allows non-traditional approaches to data collection by focusing on ensuring every voice is heard in the process. It has to address the fact that not everyone's primary form of communication is the written text and not everyone is numerate or literate (Mertens 1999).

The methodological and ideological roots of participatory evaluation lie in participatory action research (Cornwall and Jewkes 1995; Green et al. 1995). Action research is well established as an approach and methodology in many areas related to health promotion, for example in social work (Waterson 2000). Within these areas tremendous variety has been generated in the form the methodology has taken, with the approach being applied to increasingly complex problems. For example, in development research, action research has been extensively used as a vehicle for rural development and is closely associated with Freirian approaches to popular education (Rahman 1993). This southern focus, as Brown and Tandon (1983) call it, emphasises mobilisation, conscientising and empowering the oppressed to achieve community transformations and social justice – notions that have much in common with community development and empowerment for health promotion.

In management science, the notion of stakeholder and participatory evaluation is now well established (Fricke and Gill 1989) building on the notion of action research (Ragsdell 1998; Reynolds,1998) and action learning, which encourage the systematic collection of data and information, combining rigor and relevance in moving towards high levels of performance in organisations, as well as leading to innovation (Magerison 1987). The approach is geared to solving major job/organisation issues or problems on a group basis, and its focus is decision-makers. The principal investigator, the evaluator, acts as a co-ordinator of the project with responsibility for technical support training and quality control but with joint responsibility for conducting the inquiry. The evaluator becomes a partner in an evaluation process where all those involved have a commitment to change. That partnership is such that it may develop over a long period of time rather than for the duration of one project. It also means that the external contract evaluator is less likely to be co-opted or manipulated by managers in favour of their own agenda (Mathison 1994). Underpinning the rationale is the notion of learning and, more particularly, the notion of organisational learning. This reflects an increasing emphasis in management literature on the importance of participatory decision making in bringing about organisational change, and the notion of the learning organisation (Senge 1990). Transformation in organisations is seen as only taking place if the whole organisation not only monitors and evaluates operational activities but also uses that information to examine and reflect on its beliefs and values at a strategic level.

Underpinning participatory evaluation at its best are Freirian notions of critical education and praxis and action research. By encouraging people to reflect on their situation and explore what created it, a process of learning takes place. As people interrogate the information they have collected they add to collective understanding which integrates and combines all forms of knowledge through the collaborative process of inquiry. In this process new knowledge is created through dialogue as new meanings are shared and explored (Park 1999). Evaluation becomes self-directed and new avenues are explored.

A framework for the process of participatory evaluation

Like all evaluation, participatory evaluation involves a series of decision making steps. At each step, there is a set of questions or key issues that needs to be considered. These questions ensure the aims of the project and the evaluation are clear, the right objectives are set, that the correct data are collected in the right way, to measure the right outcomes in relation to the original objectives, within the resources available. At each stage, there will be choices that have to be made by the participants in the process. While the stages are described below linearly, they are part of a continual feedback cycle of reflection, planning, action and change, from setting the agenda to acting on the results. The questions that have to be answered at each stage are interrelated. So if an answer is not feasible either for political reasons, resource constraints, or lack of obtainable information, this will require a return to an earlier stage to reconsider the decisions made previously. The World Health Organization (WHO) working party on health promotion evaluation suggest the following steps:

Step 1   *Describe the proposed programme or initiative.* This includes clarifying the initiative's mandate, aims and objectives, linkage with other initiatives, procedures and structures. A programme logic model is often helpful in this process. This step will also include getting people 'on board', establishing a group to oversee and undertake the evaluation, examining the health issues of concern, and collecting baseline information.

Step 2   *Identify the issues and questions of concern for the evaluation.* This would include deciding on the purpose(s) of the evaluation, clarifying the issues that are likely to be of concern to all of the participants, including the potential users of the evaluation, and specifying evaluation questions relative to the aims and objectives of the health promotion initiative. It is important that goals and objectives of the intervention be clarified before deciding how to measure the extent to which they have been achieved. There is a danger that if ease of measurement dictates the goals or objectives, or only quantifiable objectives are pursued, a full picture is not obtained and key information is lost.

Step 3   *Design the process for obtaining the required information.* This includes deciding on the kind of evaluation to be carried out, the objects and processes to be assessed, measurement methods, which population groups and when the data are to be collected. This step should also include choosing the best approach for the questions being asked as well as a plan for implementing the design. Ensuring maximum participation in this process will ensure all experience is valued, and that information is collected from all credible sources.

Step 4   *Collect the data* by following the agreed-upon data collection methods and procedures having tested the methods through a small pilot study.

Step 5   *Analyse and evaluate the data.* This includes interpreting the data and comparing observed versus expected outcomes. It is important that all the stakeholders are involved in the process of interpretation. An example of participatory analysis is Labonte and Feather's story dialogue method (Labonte *et al.* 1999).

Step 6   *Make recommendations.* This includes clarifying short- and long-term implications of the findings, and identifying the costs and benefits of implementing and not implementing recommendations.

Step 7   *Disseminate findings.* This includes feeding back findings to funders and to other stakeholders, in a meaningful and useful form, not necessarily a report. Other ways of doing this could include posters, poems, drama or a collage.

Step 8   *Apply* what has been learnt and *take action.*

(For more details see Springett 1998)

Participants are involved in all the steps described above. The process as specified makes sure that evaluation is an integral part of the planning phase of the health promotion programme/activity as well as its management. It helps in the clarification of aims and objectives so there is a rational fit between the programme goals and activities. Considerable groundwork needs to be undertaken in clarifying what is going on and what people believe is going on. This takes time, particularly if the aim of a programme is to develop communities and where community-defined concerns need to be the focus of the programme. Indeed, since health promotion is intended to have an impact on someone either by contributing to behavioural change or changes in the environmental conditions that constrain healthy choices, then the objectives of the target group/ client themselves must be included too. Existing models and theories will inform the whole process of negotiation between stakeholders. Discussion at this stage makes explicit assumptions about causation, both those more formally validated by science as well 'lay' theories based on the unique context and everyday experience. It will be seen, therefore, that getting

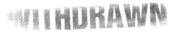

people on board at an early stage is crucial. This groundwork forms the platform for successful participatory evaluation. It will inevitably involve capacity building for all those involved and is best achieved through workshop type activities rather than formal meetings. This means engaging both professionals and the community. Acceptability of a health promotion programme needs to be established with the community. If managers are involved, the knowledge gained from evaluation is more likely to be acted upon. If funders are involved, they are more likely to understand what it has been possible to achieve in the circumstances. Even if they are not directly involved, good participatory evaluation has regular feedback from and to all those concerned as an integral part of the process. This early work is also crucial for finding out what the most appropriate programme should be and it may be that the programme is modified radically at this stage as part of the negotiation process and as people reflect on what they are trying to achieve. It is important too, where programmes are community based, that community-defined concerns drive the process of agenda setting and thus any evaluation needs to pay attention to ensuring the community voice is heard equally in the process. If the process is set up correctly then it becomes a natural and automatic review activity integral to the whole programme. This means efficient and effective data collection takes place, so small and innovative projects are not weighed down with difficult and additional claims on time and resources. By being involved, participants can see the value of the information they are collecting, which ensures greater reliability and validity. It also ensures the indicators actually measure the right things in the right way, in other words, the indicators are meaningful to all those concerned. However, the benefits of such an approach go beyond ownership and the clarity and the robustness of the data. By involving a range of people in each stage, innovative ways of measuring, process, impact and outcomes are often generated. For example, the use of digital archiving, photovoice, collage storytelling and oral history (Brinton Lykes 1998; Mienczakowski and Morgan 1998). There are no off-the-shelf methods for achieving this type of work. A common lesson, however, is that if participation falters at any stage, it is difficult for project champions to regain it at a later stage. Thus a range of techniques have to be used to generate and maintain enthusiasm and interest (Macgillavray 1998). If they are maintained, the difficult task of analysis of data and presenting it and reflecting on the lessons learnt is much easier. By taking people through the process of analysis they are much more likely to understand the information generated and also to act on the results. Here, the crucial issue is developing feedback mechanisms that go beyond the standard evaluation report that rarely gets read in its entirety. Celebration events provide an opportunity for all those who participated in collecting the data, in undertaking the project work and participating in the programmes to come together to review the lessons learnt and share their experience with others.

The nature of participatory evaluation in health promotion: two case studies

To demonstrate how participatory evaluation works this section will describe the evaluation of the Drumchapel Project in Glasgow, Scotland (Curtice *et al.* 2001) and the evaluation of the Merseyside Health Action Zone Netherton Projects (Springett and Dunkerton 2002). Both examples demonstrate the developmental role of participatory evaluation and also the social consequences of adopting such an approach.

The Drumchapel Project

The Drumchapel Project was established to test the relevance of 'health for all' principles of community participation, empowerment and collaboration in a multiply deprived community on the outskirts of Glasgow. It aimed to catalyse new ways of working among member agencies of Healthy Cities in Glasgow as well as to pilot innovative approaches to the empowerment and participation of local people through the training, recruitment and deployment of community health volunteers. The project's organisational structure and management style was also designed to maximise participation, empowerment and collaboration.

The evaluation came at the end of the two-year pilot period and was driven largely by participants' concern to pilot an evaluation method which was capable of reflecting the essence of what the project was about, namely empowerment, participation and collaboration, and of reflecting these principles in the evaluation process itself. Participants were concerned that the evaluation should contribute to the project and not the other way around. They hoped to gain something from a more appropriate evaluation in terms of new skills, a more informed perspective on the project, a stronger sense of direction, more commitment to a shared vision and a knowledge of how things could be improved. They were also keen to record and reflect upon the project's approach and achievements with a view to disseminating the practice so that they themselves and others could learn from it. At the outset of the exercise, however, many of them felt very fearful and negative about evaluation and associated it with being 'judged', 'put under a microscope' and generally scrutinised from afar by outside 'experts'.

In this evaluation, the participants' agenda took priority. The aims of the evaluation were: to explore a variety of approaches to the evaluation of the Drumchapel Healthy Cities Project; to seek the views of a range of participants as to indicators of the project's success and, to assess the feasibility of reflecting the Health For All principles of participation, empowerment and collaboration in the evaluation process. The evaluation process took place over approximately a year between November 1991 and December 1992. A variety of approaches to data collection were tried to ensure that a range of voices was heard and to give participants experience of the different methods. A questionnaire was administered to project participants to provide baseline data on their attitudes to evaluation. Training workshops were held with project participants to explore evaluation issues and introduce some qualitative methods. Over three months, a series of group meetings on evaluation were held. These meetings were the main vehicles for participation in the evaluation process and for key decision making about what should be evaluated and how. Participants appreciated the opportunity that the group meetings offered to gain an overview of the project, to exchange views with other groups and to reflect, in a group setting, on the project's progress. This illustrates the evaluation process being used to develop skills, and participation and collaboration, and not merely to collect data. Group interviews were held over a six-month period with representatives of various groups within the project. The group interviews were complemented by individual interviews with a selection of participants. In order to enable the community health volunteers to tell their own stories, case studies were prepared with them throughout May and June 1992.

A creative range of methods was employed to share the learning from the evaluation experience. These included a report and video recording the experience of undertaking a participatory approach to community health needs assessment, in which some of those people who subsequently became community health volunteers in the project had participated. A Group Art Project was run to design a tree symbolising the project. The tree symbol went on to become the cornerstone of an exhibition about the project, which was widely used in teaching and presentations. It has since been made permanent in a tile mosaic in the area's new health centre, where the project is now based. Drama was another vehicle that gave voice to the experiences of participants. One volunteer wrote a play about her experience of being a volunteer that was performed by a group of volunteers at open days and other community events. In order to look at one aspect of the project's outreach, a publicity survey was carried out by community health volunteers with support from staff to investigate the profile of the project in the community. Finally, a follow-up questionnaire was administered among project participants, in order to ascertain the level of participation in evaluation and any changes in their own attitudes and skills that they could identify as a result of the experience.

The most popular methods of evaluation were those that were creative, informal and non-threatening, and which allowed different groups within the project to exchange views. The evaluation group meetings and exercises, such as the creation of the project tree, were excellent ways of helping participants to see and appreciate the project as a whole rather than just from their own vantage point. In order for evaluation to be a participative activity, it is important that a range of approaches is adopted to maximise the chance of appealing to as many project participants as possible. Videos, exhibitions and drama are imaginative and attractive alternatives to the written word, and also have the benefit of being more attractive to the ultimate consumers of evaluation. Many people are happy to watch a play or a video, where they would be less likely to read a report. And putting together a video or performing a play tends to be a collective activity in a way that writing a report is not.

As little as possible was decided in advance so that the evaluation process was left free to evolve in negotiation with participants. The evaluation process was useful to participants in developing new insights into the project, clarifying and refining its organisational structure and direction, and identifying weaknesses as well as strategies to rectify them. The before-and-after questionnaires demonstrated a significant shift in attitudes to evaluation, with the original fear factor almost completely absent and a very high value being placed on evaluation across all categories of participants. The only concern repeatedly expressed was that the time spent on evaluation should not be to the detriment of sustaining the practice. Capacity building for evaluation was a key feature of the process and this allowed a more outcome-focused approach to the next stage, with project participants no longer afraid of evaluation and equipped with the skills and confidence to ensure integration of evaluation and practice.

Merseyside Health Action Zone Netherton Projects

In Merseyside Health Action Zone (MHAZ) a participatory action research approach to evaluation framework development for projects was adopted within a set of broader principles-driven Zone wide framework. The aim was to ensure that evaluation would generate knowledge for use locally but also at policy level and contribute to sustainable learning systems. Learning and evaluation were identified as key elements in the 'Making It Happen' stream of the MHAZ implementation plan (Merseyside Health Action Zone 2000). As part of the six-monthly performance monitoring requirements, HAZ-funded projects were asked to provide evidence of how what they are doing contributed to the seven HAZ principles (Cropper 2001a). To support projects, an evaluation training programme was put in place. This training programme was rolled out at all levels of the HAZ, from strategic level right down to community level. The training programme encouraged a participatory evaluation approach with the focus on learning through evaluation. All MHAZ work is principles-driven and evaluation is no exception (Cropper 2001b). The local evaluation has, therefore, devised a framework that supports local learning and it is one that encourages participatory evaluation while promoting a consistent approach to evaluation across the HAZ. Merseyside HAZ was also being evaluated by the National Evaluation Team of the Health Action Zone (Springett and Young 2002). This team used a 'Theory of Change' approach to evaluation and this approach was incorporated into the local evaluation framework, thus linking programme into policy at all levels.

The Aspen Institute in the United States first developed the Theories of Change (ToC) approach (Connell *et al.* 1995). It is an approach that was specifically developed to address the complex nature of community-based social interventions and therefore has much to offer health promotion evaluation. In a ToC approach, evaluators work with participants to identify the variety of potential theories of change that stakeholders hold about what they expect the consequences of the actions they propose will be. It allows participants to explore their own assumptions about the way change will take place. It also encourages the elaboration of the context in which projects are working. This enables projects to see what could be realistically undertaken within both resource constraints and the context in which they are working. It therefore encourages a form of critical reflection on why they are doing what they are doing as well as giving equal value to lay and ' expert' theories of change. Once the theories have been articulated and a form of consensus achieved, the theories of change are encapsulated in a plan which is used as a framework for data collection. An essential element of the approach is that these plans are not set in concrete but are revisited by projects and programmes each year and, in the light of the data collected and of experience, changed where appropriate, thus responding to the fluidity of the change process. On the other hand, a ToC approach also introduces greater rigour into project planning. An additional benefit is that it encourages participants in short-term projects to see themselves as part of a bigger picture, both in relation to broader programmes of which they are part and of the social context. By making explicit the context, one also ensures that if changes in the context occur, there is an explicit framework for recording those changes and ensuring that such a change was taken into account in assessing project outcomes. This encourages the type of recording and observation that enables unexpected outcomes to be captured and local knowledge to be incorporated into the evaluation. Making the assumptions and theories of project participants explicit, both to themselves and their co-workers, has been found also to be useful where there is a rapid turnover of staff (Springett and Young 2002).

One of the earliest Merseyside Health Action Zone projects to be funded was a participatory evaluation of a set of HAZ/Urban Projects in Netherton, an area of Sefton Borough, which is a deprived outer estate on the fringes of the Merseyside conurbation. The evaluation was spearheaded by the Netherton Partnership which itself was funded by the Single Regeneration Fund. The uniqueness of the approach was that it both provided a pilot for the implementation of good practice in evaluation within the Zone, and it brought together a set of projects for the purposes of evaluation within an area (Springett and Dunkerton 2001). Also, with a view to capacity building, they were supported through the process with training.

An initial one-day workshop took place in March 2000 and this brought the projects together for the first time. The workshop introduced a process of participatory evaluation drawing on the WHO Guidance on the evaluation of health promotion (Springett 1998). Following the workshop, a steering group was elected and two further two-hour meetings took place. It was during this period of initial engagement with the process of evaluation that the participants were asked to clarify their theories of change using specially created forms based on the framework developed by the national evaluation team. Projects then peer reviewed in groups each others' ToCs and these were revised. Although most projects subsequently reported that the process had been useful, there was some initial resistance to this approach as many felt it was either too linear for the types of projects they were engaging in or too long-term for short two-year projects. Some of the resistance stemmed from confusing monitoring with evaluation. When discussions started, however, on how they were going to demonstrate the achievement of their aims and objectives, the realisation dawned that evaluation was more than number crunching and had real potential for creative ideas and for the collection of information through a variety of other media, including video, art and celebration days. These are tools that are integral to project development, particularly with marginalised and socially excluded groups who often have a low level of literacy. It was at this point that the projects took ownership of the evaluation and a creative process emerged that combined learning with doing.

Ownership was a key to change in attitude and to an ongoing emergent and iterative process of evaluation development. Bringing projects together generated a broader focus and encouraged the sharing of resources and ideas. Discussion highlighted a common concern for collecting information on confidence and self-worth, income security, quality of life and community well-being. When the projects took the lead in developing both the evaluation framework and training, the training focused on success, fun and celebration as a vehicle for evaluation. Participants felt that the aim of evaluation should be to capture the 'lived experience' of the projects and their impact on people's lives. Monthly two-hour meetings enabled participants, in collaboration with others, to work through in greater depth the issues raised in the initial workshop and meetings, and to support each other in evaluation. Thus the early resistance disappeared and enthusiasm for evaluation emerged. It came to be seen as a natural activity integral to the project rather than a burden. In May 2001 a celebration day was held in a marquee in the main centre of Netherton. All twelve projects had a stall or display to demonstrate their achievements and outcomes, and activities in which people could participate. There was face-painting for children and a local artist painted a collage of the day. This celebratory approach to evaluation was also followed by MHAZ as a whole. In October of the same year all the projects within the HAZ were brought together in one location for a day. The aim was to provide information on what they were doing to share with others. In the morning they were given an opportunity to evaluate each other's project and in the afternoon the event was open to the general public. Participants reported that this was a very effective way to encourage them to record the process and outcomes of their work as peer pressure to demonstrate progress provided the motivation to succeed (Chendo Thomas, personal communication).

Towards a values-and-principles driven approach to knowledge development through evaluation

To be of real use evaluation should contribute to the development of knowledge of what works and what does not work in particular contexts and under particular conditions. It should not be undertaken in a manner that actually undermines the process and values of the projects being evaluated. The two examples discussed here come from programmes committed to community and practitioner involvement in decision-making and capacity building. Building evaluation into project development in a way that encourages learning has been a key feature. Both participatory evaluation and theories of change approaches ensure evaluation is built into project planning and development in a way that conventional evaluation does not. By combining both participatory and theories of change approaches, a more people-orientated approach to targets and outcome setting emerges, which allows those targets and outcomes to change in the light of circumstances. Both approaches go some way to addressing issues of relationship, complexity and change that lie at the heart of promoting health, while at the same time ensuring that evaluation and health promotion practice is empowering in itself. What is very clear is that when projects and communities determine their own theories of change and aims and objectives, the focus is not on disease and illness, but on well-being and quality of life.

Recent demands for evidence-based practice have put pressure on those committed to health promotion approaches to justify the effectiveness of their practice and to demonstrate measurable outcomes. Internationally it has resulted in a number of initiatives, particularly in the Americas and Europe, which aim to build an 'evidence base' for health promotion. Although in the process of the development of these initiatives there have been debates on what constitutes evidence in health promotion (McQueen 2000; McQueen and Anderson 2001) and the criteria by which evidence is defined have been subject to philosophical and theoretical scrutiny (Wiggers and Sanson-Fisher 1998), there remains a danger that initiatives will encourage the very value systems they seek to challenge by buying into the notion of the existence of objective evidence. This will divert limited resources from knowledge development to collecting evidence to satisfy a managerial agenda driven by searches for efficiency, cost effectiveness and quality assurance in public expenditure, which, in the UK at least, has led to an obsession with targets and indicators. Much better that those resources are invested in the development of approaches which address the complex holistic nature of the social change processes that constitute health promotion. It is also important that the methods and criteria of effectiveness used are consistent with the fundamental principles of health promotion, empowerment, participation, collaboration and equity.

One international initiative which has done this is that which has been spearheaded by PAHO in the Americas (Pan-American Health Organization 2000). The initiative has developed a series of principles concerning the evaluation of 'health municipalities'. These have been called the Antigua Principles. These principles have formed the basis of an evaluation framework that is being implemented at various locations in the Americas using a common workbook. It is this framework that will drive the evidence collected through a local participatory process. In this way both the local and general knowledge base will be enhanced and developed without undermining local development trajectories or undermining the spirit of health promotion. This unique transcultural endeavour should be replicated elsewhere.

Given the increasing inequalities in health, it is the nature of the work of health promotion that it involves working with disempowered and marginalised groups. As argued at the beginning of this chapter, changing the power relations so excluded groups can have a say and 'take control' of the factors that create health lies at the heart of health promotion. The most appropriate type of evaluation, therefore, is one that involves enhancing this control through critical reflection and learning (Vanderplaat 1995). As John Ruskin once wrote, the only real and lasting transformation comes through freeing people's thinking and values (Landow 1985: 85).

References

Brinton Lykes, M. (1998) 'Creative Arts and Photography in Participatory Action Research in Guatemala', in P. Reason and H. Bradbury *A Handbook of Action Research*. London: Sage, pp. 363–70.

Brooks, J.G. and Brooks, M.G. (1993) *In Search of Understanding: The Case for Constructivist Classrooms*. Alexandria, VA: Association for Supervision & Curriculum Development.

Brown, L.D. and Tandon, R. (1983) Ideology and Political Economy in Inquiry: Action Research and Participatory Action Research', *Journal of Applied Behavioural Science* 3: 277–94.

Brown, J.S., Collins, A. and Duguid, P. (1995) *Situated Cognition and the Culture of Learning*. Institute for Learning Technologies

Chen, H.T. (1990) *Theory-Driven Evaluations*. Thousand Oaks, CA: Sage.

Connell, J.P., Kubisch, A.C., Schorr, L.B. and Weiss, C.H. (ed.) (1995) *New Approaches to Evaluating Community Initiatives: Concepts Methods and Contexts*. Washington, DC: Aspen Institute.

Cornwall, A. and Jewkes, R. 'What is Participatory Research?' *Social Science and Medicine* 41(12): 1667–76.

Cranton, Patricia (1996). *Professional Development as Transformative Learning*. San Francisco: Jossey-Bass.

Cropper, A. (2001a) *Evaluation Handbook for Health Action Zone Funded Interventions in Merseyside*.

Cropper, A. (2001b) *Learning from Change: An Evaluation Strategy for Merseyside Health Action Zone*.

Curtice, L., Springett, J. and Kennedy, A. (2001) 'Evaluation in Urban Settings: The Challenge of Healthy Cities', in I. Rootman *et al.* (eds) *Evaluation in Health Promotion: Principles and Perspectives.* Copenhagen: WHO/Euro.

Everitt, A. (1996) 'Values and Evidence in Evaluating Community Health', *Critical Public Health* 6(3): 56–65.

Fawcett, S.B. *et al.* (2001) 'Evaluating Community Initiatives for Health and Development', in I. Rootman *et al.* (eds) *Evaluation in Health Promotion: Principles and Perspectives*, WHO Regional Publication series no. 92. Copenhagen: WHO.

Frankish, C.J., Milligan, C.D. and Reid, C. (1998) 'A Review of Relationships Between Active Living and Determinants of Health', *Social Science and Medicine* 47(3): 287–301.

Freire, P. (1976) *Education: The Practice of Freedom.* London: Writers and Readers.

Fricke, J.G. and Gill, R. (1989) 'Participative Evaluation', *Canadian Journal of Program Evaluation* 4(1): 11–25.

Garanta, J. (1993) 'The Powerful, the Powerless and the Experts, Knowledge Struggles in an Information Age', in P. Park, M. Brydon-Miller, B. Hall and T. Jackson (eds) *Voices of Change: Participatory Research in the United States and Canada.* Toronto: Oise Press.

Glouberman, S. (2000) 'A Dynamic Concept of Health', in *Towards a New Concept of Health*, CPRN Discussion Paper H/03 August.

Goodman, R.M., Wheeler, F. C. and P.R. Lee (1993) 'Evaluation of the Heart to Heart Project: Lessons from a Community Based Chronic Disease Prevention Programme', *American Journal of Health Promotion* 9(6): 443–55.

Graham, H. (1998) 'Promoting Health against Inequality: Using Research to Identify Targets for Intervention – A Case Study of Women and Smoking', *Health Education Journal* 57(4): 292–302.

Green, L.W. *et al.* (1995)*The Royal Society of Canada Study of Participatory Research in Health Promotion.* University of British Columbia.

Greene, J.C. (1994) 'Qualitative Program Evaluation, Practice and Promise', in N.K. Denzin and Y.S. Lincoln (eds) *Handbook of Qualitative Research.* Thousand Oaks, CA: Sage.

Gustavsen, B. (1992) *Dialogue and Development.* Assen : Van Gorcum.

Henkel, M. (1991) 'The New Evaluative State', *Public Administration* 69: 121–36.

Kolb, D.A. (1984) *Experiential Learning: Experience as a Source of Learning and Development.* Englewood Cliffs, NJ: Prentice Hall.

Kushner, S. (2000) *Personalizing Evaluation.* London: Sage.

Labonte, R. (1994) 'Health Promotion and Empowerment: Reflections on Professional Practice', *Health Education Quarterly* 21(2): 253–68.

Labonte, R. (1999) 'Health Promotion in the Near Future: Remembrances of Activism Past', *Health Education Journal* 58(4): 365–77.

Labonte, R., Feather, J. and Hills, M. (1999) 'A Story Dialogue Method for Health Promotion Knowledge Development and Evaluation', *Health Education Research* 14(1): 39–50.

Landow, G.P. (1985) *John Ruskin.* OUP.

Loughlin, K. (1996) 'Learning to Change: New Dimensions', *Australian Journal of Adult and Community Education* 36(1): 54–63.

Macgillavray, A. (1998) 'Turning the Sustainable Corner :How to Indicate Right', in D. Warburton (ed.) *Community and Sustainable Development, Participation for the Future*. London: Earthscan, pp. 81–95.

McQueen, D.V. (2000) *Strengthening the Evidence Base for Health Promotion: A Report on Evidence for the Fifth Global Conference on Health Promotion*. Mexico City, 5–9 June. Geneva: WHO.

McQueen, D.V. and Anderson, L. (2001) 'What Counts as Evidence? Issues and Debates on Evidence Relevant to the Evaluation of Community Health Promotion Programs', in I. Rootman *et al.* (eds) *Evaluation in Health Promotion: Principles and Perspectives*. Copenhagen: WHO/Euro.

Magerison, C.J. (1987) 'Integrating Action Research and Action Learning in Organisational Development', *Organisational Development* winter: 88–91.

Mathison, S. (1994) 'Rethinking the Evaluator Role : Partnerships between Organisations and Evaluators', *Evaluation and Planning* 17(3): 299–304.

Merseyside Health Action Zone (MHAZ) (2000) *MHAZ Implementation Plan*.

Mertens, D. (1999) 'Inclusive Evaluation: Implications of Transformative Theory for Evaluation', *American Journal of Evaluation* 20(1): 1–14.

Mienczakowski, J. and Morgan, S. (1998) 'Ethnodrama: Constructing Participatory, Experiential and Compelling Action Research through Performance', in P. Reason and H. Bradbury (eds) *A Handbook of Action Research*. London: Sage, pp. 219–26.

Nutbeam, D. (1998) 'Evaluating Health Promotion – Progress, Problems and Solutions', *Health Promotion International* 13: 27–44.

Park, P. (1999) 'People, Knowledge and Change in Participatory Research', *Management Learning* 30(2): 141–57.

Pawson, R. and Tilley, N. (1998) *Realistic Evaluation*. London: Sage.

Peile, C. (1994) 'Theory, Practice, Research: Casual Acquaintances or a Seamless Whole?', *Australian Social Work* 47(2): 17–23.

Raeburn, J. and Rootman, I. (1998) *People-Centred Health Promotion*. London: Wiley.

Ragsdell, G. (1998) 'Participatory Action Research and the Development of Critical Creativity: A "Natural Combination"', *Systemic Practice and Action Research* 11(1): 508–15.

Rahman, M.A. (1993) *People's Self-Development: Perspectives on Participatory Action Research*. London: Zed Books.

Reynolds, M. (1998) 'Reflection and Critical Reflection in Management Learning', *Management Learning* 29(2): 184–99.

Seddon, J. (2000) 'On Target to Nothing', *The Observer* 27 Aug.: 36.

Senge, P. (1990) *The Fifth Discipline: The Art and the Practice of Organisational Learning*. New York: Doubleday.

Shephard, P. (1996) 'Worksite Fitness and Exercise Programs: A Review of Methodology and Health Impact', *American Journal of Health Promotion* 10(6): 436–52.

South, J. and Tilford, S. (2000) 'Perceptions of Research and Evaluation in Health Promotion Practice and Influences on Activity', *Health Education Research Theory and Practice* 15(6): 729–41.

Springett, J. (1998) *Practical Guidance on Evaluating Health Promotion*. Copenhagen: WHO/Euro.

Springett, J. (2001) 'Appropriate Approaches for the Evaluation of Health Promotion', *Critical Public Health* 11(2): 139–51.

Springett, J. and Dunkerton, L. (2002) *HAZ/Netherton Evaluation Report*. Liverpool: Institute for Health, Liverpool John Moores University.

Springett, J. and Leavey, C. (1995) 'Participatory Action Research, the Development of a Paradigm: Dilemmas and Prospects', in N. Bruce, J. Springett, J. Hodgkiss and A. Scott Samuel (eds) *Research and Change in Urban Community Health*. Aldershot: Avebury, pp. 57–66.

Springett, J. and Young, A. (2002) 'Comparing Theories of Change and Participatory Approaches to the Evaluation of Projects within Health Action Zones: Two Views from the North West on Engaging Community Level Projects in Evaluation', in L. Baud and K. Judge (eds) *Learning from Health Action Zones*. Chichester: Aeneas Press.

Van Eyk, H., Baum, F. and Blandford, J. (2001) 'Evaluating Healthcare Reform: The Challenge of Evaluating Changing Policy', *Evaluation* 7(4) 487–503.

Vanderplaat, M. (1995) 'Beyond Technique: Issues in Evaluating for Empowerment', *Evaluation* 1(1): 81–96.

Wallerstein, N. (1999) 'Power between Evaluator and Community: Research Relationships within New Mexico's Healthier Communities', *Social Science and Medicine* 49(1): 39–53.

Wallerstein, N. and Bernstein, E. (1994) 'Empowerment Education: Freire's Ideas Adapted to Health Education', *Health Education Quarterly* 15(4): 379–394.

Wallerstein, N. and Freudenberg, N. (1998) 'Linking Health Promotion and Social Justice: A Rationale and Two Case Stories', *Health Education Research* 13(3): 451–7.

Waterson, J. (2000) 'Balancing Research and Action: Reflections on an Action Research Project in a Social Services Department', *Social Policy ad Administration* 34(4): 494–508.

Watkins, K.E. and Marsick, V.J. (1992) 'Towards a Theory of Informal and Incidental Learning in Organizations', *International Journal of Lifelong Education* 2(4).

Weiss, C.H. (1988) 'Evaluation for Decisions: Is There Anybody There? Does Anybody Care?', *Education Practice* 9: 15–20.

Wiggers, J. and Sanson-Fisher, R. (1998) 'Evidence-Based Health Promotion', in D. Scott and R. Weston (eds) *Evaluating Health Promotion*. Cheltenham, UK: Thornes.

Williams, G. and Popay, J. (1994) 'Lay Knowledge and the Privilege of Experience', in J. Gabe, D. Kelleher and G. Williams (eds) *Challenging Medicine*. London: Routledge.

Wood, S. and Lake, J. (2000) *Second Report on the Evaluation of Merseyside Smoking Cessation Programme*. Institute for Health; Liverpool John Moores University.

Woods, S.E., Lake, J.R. and Springett, J. (in press) 'Tackling Health Inequalities and the HAZ Smoking Cessation Programme: The Perfect Match?', *Critical Public Health*.

World Health Organisation (1986) *The Ottawa Charter for Health Promotion*. Geneva: WHO.

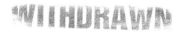

Index

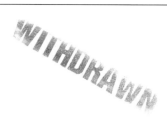

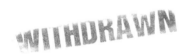